Chair Yoga for Seniors

The Guide for Strong and Flexible Body

Jannah Adams

professional before attempting any techniques outlined in this book.

By reading this document, the reader agrees that under no circumstances is the author responsible for any losses, direct or indirect, that are incurred as a result of the use of the information contained within this document, including, but not limited to, errors, omissions, or inaccuracies.

Table of Contents

Introduction

Aging is not lost youth but a new stage of opportunity and strength. —Frank Lloyd Wright

It is a blessing to get older. The wisdom, experience, lessons, and years of adventure that we have experienced should not be lost on us. And whilst we can celebrate the years we have under our belt, there is also a bittersweet element to aging as we begin to experience certain physical changes that we cannot ignore.

I am here to tell you that this does not have to be. We may be changing physically, but it is not too late to invest in our physical health and ensure we live out the rest of our years filled with well-being and good vitality.

Believe me, I know what it is like when you feel your mobility is not what it used to be. I have been in situations where I have questioned my strength and stability. And there have been times when I have questioned my body image.

Do you know what got me through those moments? My yoga practice.

There are approximately 300 million practicing yogis who can be found across the world. This is not surprising since yoga is very accessible and speaks to all genders and ages. You can find a yoga studio in almost every city in every country, which has contributed to its growth globally (Drah, 2020).

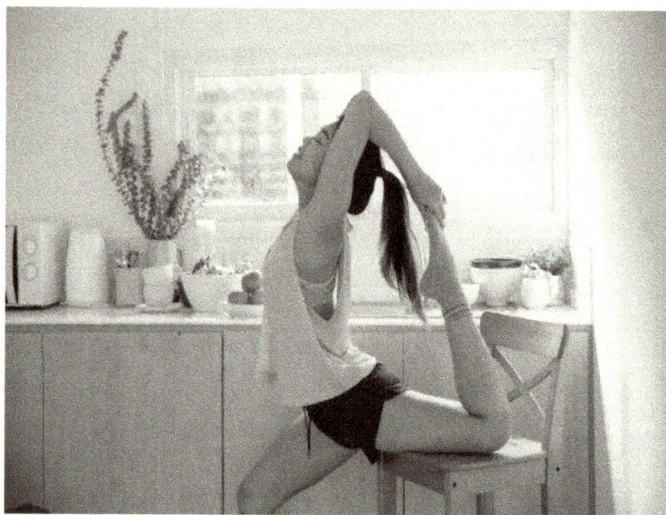

Research from 2016 has shown that in the United States alone, the number of yoga practitioners has gone up from 20.4 million to 36 million, so it is safe to assume that this number has increased substantially (Galic, 2022).

One of the biggest attractions of yoga is the physical benefits it provides for us, regardless of age. The statistics and research below illustrate the benefits of practicing yoga.

Data from Galic (2022) shows that 20% of practitioners have a better sense of mobility, strength, and flexibility compared to nonpractitioners. The reason that most people start yoga is that they are concerned about their flexibility, stress levels, overall health, and general fitness. They believe yoga can help them with those concerns—and they are right.

We cannot fight aging, but we can make the years that are going to pass some of the best years of our lives. Society paints aging in a negative light, and we are constantly bombarded with images and narratives about frailty and the idea that we lose our independence when we get older. It does not have to be this way. It is not too late to take back control of your physical health and combat these common concerns.

I realize that suddenly it seems that your body is working against you. What used to come easy now takes a bit more work. Mobility is one of those issues. Joints may seem stiffer, muscles less responsive, and movement stifled.

The lack or decrease of physical movement is one of the main culprits, and I often see that this lack of activity turns into a vicious cycle. You stop moving because it feels uncomfortable, but movement begins to feel uncomfortable because you stop moving, and thus it continues in this way until you cease all sorts of activity. You stop feeling strong and capable, which impacts your motivation to take care of yourself physically.

Other mobility issues can stem from not just a lack of activity but also poor nutrition. As we get older, we tend to care less about what we are eating, especially if we are living by ourselves and eating alone. We may not have the capacity to cook nutritious meals daily.

Secondly, in terms of biology, our metabolism changes as well as our nutritional needs, and we often do not adapt our nutrition to keep up with these differences.

Is there any good news? I apologize for the negativity, but these are the facts, and I am pleased to say that there is good news. According to The National Centre for Complementary and Integrative Health (2015), yoga motivated people to incorporate other forms of exercise into their daily routines as well as encouraged them to relook at their eating habits and adopt better nutritional lifestyles.

I will be honest, aging has taken its toll on me mentally, and I do find myself reminiscing about my past physical capabilities, especially when it comes to areas of my life where I may be more reliant on strength. I know that I may have been more agile and in better health a couple of years ago, but my yoga practice has staved off most of my bigger concerns.

Those concerns are that I will lose my independence and have to rely on other people as I get older. I understand that worry; most seniors are afraid of becoming a burden on their families. You do not have to resign yourself to that narrative. I am going to show you how to maintain your independence, build and hold onto your strength, work on your mobility and flexibility, and boost your self-esteem.

I know it may seem daunting to start a new exercise regime, but you cannot deny that now is the best time to start. You would not have picked up this book if you did not believe that. I am glad that you can no longer ignore the benefits exercise has for your well-being and longevity, and that is what I am going to do.

I am going to make it as easy as possible for you. You are going to get a program that provides you with stretches, movements, and poses to work on your balance and mobility. It will help you build a strong core and increase your strength and overall fitness. Your balance will improve, and your risk of falling will reduce. Your joints and muscles will benefit from the stretching and mobility, helping you relieve aches and pains.

You can do this program in the comfort of your home, and all you will need is a chair. My goal is to provide you with accessible exercise so you can live a healthier and happier life.

I have seen how frustrated my various friends and family members become when establishing a health and fitness routine, especially when starting later in life. I believe that it does not need to be so complicated. All you require is simple at-home workouts coupled with delicious home-cooked food as the key to living a high-quality life. I have dedicated a great many years of research and practical applications in this field to provide you with this resource.

Yoga—and chair yoga, which is a more refined and accessible form of yoga—will help you craft the rest of your days as ones that are filled with well-being and longevity. From CEOs, sports teams, musicians, and actors—yoga has become the go-to practice to improve physical, mental, and spiritual health.

I am looking forward to starting this journey with you.

Part One: Understanding

Yoga... and You

Chapter 1:

A Run Down on Aging

Aging is inevitable, and there is nothing we can do to fight the progress of time. We can only do what is in our power to ensure that those years are as healthy as we can make them and live our years comfortably without the physical limitations that come from the process.

Our bodies are not built to age, and there have been very rare instances of people who have lived lives well past the 100-year mark, one of those being Frenchwoman Jeanne Calmet who passed away at age 122. It seems that our body's "set point" in terms of aging is around 90 years of age. Anything past that and you have had a very long life.

I must admit I have never looked at aging from a biological angle. I always saw it as a part of life that comes about as time progresses. I never asked *why* we age. According to Monica Menesini, aging occurs when the interactions between our bodies and elements, such as our diet and sunlight and toxins found in our environment, cause changes within our bodies (TED-

Ed, 2016). The changes occur in our cells and molecules and lead to their decline.

Surprisingly, aging is very misunderstood, and scientists are still working on how the mechanics of it work. What we do know is that, as we grow older, the DNA and cells in our bodies are damaged. When we experience this genetic damage, our cells begin to lose the ability to regenerate and function properly. This occurs with a group of cells called mitochondria, which is a cell that creates the main energy source that helps the other cells in our bodies function optimally. The knock-on effect of the decline in the function of mitochondria is that other cells cannot do their jobs efficiently and deteriorate, thus creating a chain reaction where whole organs eventually deteriorate as well.

Cellular degeneration is a fact of life, and as we continue to get older, our biological processes work against us, and we will age. Whilst we cannot counteract this, we can do things that set us up for longevity and place us in a position to age well.

What are some of the symptoms of aging? What can you expect?

Common Physical Changes as We Age

According to the World Health Organization (2022), more people are living longer than ever before. They have identified that we are currently seeing that, in each country, the older demographic is experiencing a growth surge in both size and proportion of older people in those particular populations.

They claim that by 2030, approximately one in six people will be over the age of 60, and by 2050 the number of people aged 60 will double (World Health Organization, 2022).

And all of us are connected in that we are bound to go through some changes physically as we age. These changes usually start to become more apparent as we hit our 30s and we begin to notice a slight decline in our physical and mental capacities.

We can expect changes to our cardiovascular system, digestive system, bladder, and urinary tract, memory and thinking skills, eyes and ears, teeth, skin, weight and bones, joints, and muscles.

Heart Health

As you get older, your cardiovascular system begins to change. According to WebMD Editorial Contributors (2021), it becomes harder for your heart to pump blood around your body as your arteries begin to stiffen. This added strain on your heart causes your resting heart to rise and elevate, which can lead to high blood pressure and other heart-related diseases.

Your heart rate will also stay elevated long after you exercise, making your recovery more taxing on your body.

Digestive System

Along with your cardiovascular system, your digestive system will also begin to change. This is particularly noticeable with your large intestine. Your food takes longer to digest as it moves through your digestive system slower. Your stomach, liver, small intestine, and pancreas also produce fewer digestive juices.

These changes often lead to an increase in constipation issues. These problems with bowel movements can also be attributed to certain medications you may be taking, lack of exercise, and dehydration. So remember to move, exercise, and drink enough water.

Urinary Tract and Bladder

As we age, our muscles weaken. The pelvic floor, which is a muscle that holds up our organs, such as our bladder and uterus, weakens as well. This weakening of the pelvic floor can lead to urinary and bladder discomfort as it becomes difficult to empty your bladder. Your bladder may also become less elastic, which increases your urge to urinate.

Cognitive Function, Thinking Skills, and Memory

Common complaints amongst those who are getting older are that their memories and cognitive functions are not quite what they used to be. There are often reports of forgetfulness and trouble with simple recall, and some people may find multitasking more difficult than before.

As you age, the nerves found in your spine and brain decrease, and we begin to lose the connection between them as our neural pathways change. We also see the development of plaques and tangles, which are abnormal growths that occur in the brain.

Eyesight and Hearing

Our eyesight can deteriorate as we get older, which is a normal and very common occurrence. Some symptoms are that you may struggle to see and focus on things that are close to you, you may find it difficult to see in the dark, or you may even begin to develop cataracts.

Along with diminishing eyesight, you may also experience a decline in hearing. This is due to several physical changes that occur within the ear. As time goes by, we find that our eardrums become thicker and the walls of our ear canals get thinner, making hearing more of a challenge.

Teeth

Tooth infections and decay may increase as you age. Certain medications, such as blood pressure and cholesterol medication, can contribute to dry mouth and cause discomfort. Some changes occur to your gums as they begin to pull away from your teeth.

Skin

Dryness, thinness, and fragility are all changes that occur with our skin as we age. We lose oil and elasticity, and you may develop harmless skin tags as well. You are also more prone to bruising and may notice an increase in age spots and, of course, wrinkles.

Weight

Weight gain may occur as your metabolism starts to decline and your daily activity lessens.

Bones, Joints, and Muscles

Bones become less dense as we age, which can increase your chance of fractures as they become weaker. Your connective tissue, such as cartilage, begins to weaken. Muscles will also lose strength and endurance, and you may find yourself becoming less flexible. These changes can also impact your stability, balance, and coordination.

Sex Life

As a man and woman, your sex life will change as your body ages. Women usually experience less arousal as vaginal dryness occurs, making intercourse more painful. Men usually experience impotence.

I would just like to pause here briefly as I am sure that all this information is rather overwhelming, and, as seniors, we may feel like we are faced with quite the uphill battle. I want to assure you that we can set ourselves up to live the rest of our years comfortably by taking action now.

It is not too late to change our path toward health and well-being. This book is your first step in that direction.

Your exercise routine and diet are two tools that you can use to effect great change. Keep that in mind as we continue. We are not bound by our genes. While they play a big role in the aging process, we can use tools that are in our control to change our aging process.

Our physical and social environments play a very important role in this next chapter of our lives, and if we are aware of this, we can create environments that support aging well.

We need to take a holistic look at our lives and adapt each area to create deep health, which is not reliant on only our physical well-being.

Common Health Issues

As we age and experience some of the physical changes listed above, we may also find ourselves at greater risk for certain age-related diseases.

Alzheimer's Disease

Alzheimer's disease is characterized by forgetting recently learned information, having to consistently be told new information, the need for memory aids, confusion about times and places, and having to rely on other people with certain tasks that they may not be able to perform currently.

Alzheimer's is one of the most common dementia ailments among senior citizens and there is no cure, only treatment and management. Certain factors can heighten your risk of developing dementia, such as substance abuse, depression, hypertension, and diabetes (National Institute on Aging, n.d.-d).

Arthritis

Arthritis is a painful disease that can impact our quality of life as we get older. It is a disease that affects the joints, tissue around the joints, as well as connective tissue.

According to the Centers for Disease Control and Prevention (2021), there are over 100 different types of arthritis, with specific symptoms varying according to the type of arthritis. Although there is no cure, it can be successfully treated and managed.

Depression

The World Health Organization (2017) states that over 15% of people over the age of 60 suffer from a mental health disorder. While grief is a normal part of life and is usually experienced during major life events, such as death, loss of income, or poor health, depression is not a normal part of growing older and can impact your standard of living substantially.

This often results in symptoms being overlooked and not taken seriously. Thankfully, there are many ways that you can get help and alleviate your symptoms.

Diabetes

Diabetes occurs when your body has difficulty processing sugar, and it is considered a lifestyle disease. We have seen an increase in obesity amongst older populations, which has resulted in a rise in diabetes rates (Jaul & Barron, 2017). Diabetes is a disease that can lead to other complications, such as cardiovascular diseases. It is also a disease that requires a lot of self-management, which may become troublesome as we get older.

Ensuring that you eat healthily and get enough exercise are two ways to lessen your chances of developing diabetes as you get older.

Fall Related Injuries

As mentioned previously, physical changes may result in a loss of balance and stability, which can increase our risk of falling. Falls can lead to fractures, broken bones, and abrasions, so it is important to lessen the chances of falling and hurting ourselves.

There are some precautions you can take, such as making sure you have enough Vitamin D, maintaining a balance-based exercise following an exercise routine, and ensuring that your surroundings at home are safe.

Falls account for over half of the injuries experienced by older members of society and can easily be avoided by taking the right precautions (Jaul & Barron, 2017).

At the end of every chair yoga practice, I have included balance exercises to guide you and help you resist this factor of aging.

Heart Disease

Cardiovascular disease is the leading cause of death among older populations (Jaul & Barron, 2017). The most common disease is atherosclerosis, which is a condition where fatty deposits and plaque fill up the walls of the arteries. Atherosclerosis can then lead to a long list of other cardiac issues such as heart attacks or strokes.

Influenza

The older we are, the more at risk we are for developing complications due to influenza. Our risk for hospitalization rises because our immune system weakens as we age, leaving us more vulnerable to catching the flu and less able to successfully defend ourselves against it.

Oral Health

Good oral hygiene is of particular focus as we get older as our teeth and gums begin to deteriorate. The effect this can have on our quality of life is quite profound as it affects eating as well as communication.

Issues such as unintended weight loss, dehydration, malnutrition, pain, and digestive problems can occur due to poor oral health. Keep up your dental plan and see your dentist regularly.

Osteoarthritis

Osteoarthritis is a common source of pain and disability amongst the older population. Although research has shown that it is more common among females, males need to be just as attentive and be screened by their healthcare providers (Jaul & Barron, 2017).

Exercise is a great tool to counteract this as obesity is one of the leading factors in developing osteoarthritis, particularly in the knees and hips.

It is wise to manage your bone density and potential bone loss as you get older, and this disease can be managed with medication as well as surgery.

Pneumonia

Pneumonia is an infection of the lungs. Most pneumonia cases are caused by viruses but can also be caused by other microorganisms, such as fungi and bacteria. You are more susceptible to pneumonia if you drink alcohol, have asthma, an immune disorder, or heart disease.

According to Schein (2018), pneumonia is the eighth leading cause of death in America.

Shingles

Shingles are a part of the same family of viruses that cause chickenpox. It is a very painful rash that lasts a couple of weeks and is characterized by blisters on the skin.

Our weakened immune system cannot fight off the virus, but it often occurs just once and then does not reoccur. Other factors that contribute to our susceptibility to catching shingles are stress, injury, and certain medications.

Ways Around Aging by Taking Care of Our Bodies

Creating habits and processes to aid you in aging well does not need to be complicated or costly. There are simple actions you can take that will help you create a lifestyle that sets you up for years of good health and well-being.

We will take a look at some of these tools you can use to reduce your chances of experiencing any of the complaints listed previously. These are all actions that you can take to improve your physical health; we will move on to our mental health later in the chapter.

Physical Activity

I am sure that I do not need to explain how much I believe that physical activity is one of the prominent actions you can take to help you lead a more fulfilling life. I did create a book around movement after all.

Not only do I want you to delay any aging-related problems, but I also want you to grow stronger as you age. I do not believe that we are just required to maintain our current fitness and health but also to improve it. It is never too late, and I know that this idea is one most people are susceptible to believing. The idea is to understand that any activity is better than no activity at all.

According to guidelines from the Centers for Disease Control and Prevention (n.d.-a), adults over 65 years of age should aim for three different forms of exercise.

They should be aiming for 150 minutes a week of moderate-intensity activity. They can break this down into five 30-minute exercises a week, such as brisk walking. Alternatively, they could do 75 minutes of vigorous-intensity activity, which includes hiking, jogging, or running.

You can gauge your intensity by using a scale of perceived exertion where zero is sitting and ten is working as hard as you are able. The moderate intensity would be classified as a five. You will also be able to hold a conversation but not be able to sing.

Vigorous activity will sit on a scale of around seven or eight. Your heart rate will be high, and you will need to stop to catch your breath if you're trying to speak.

Please remember that this is also very relative as we are all in different places within our fitness journeys. One person's walk may be considered another person's form of vigorous activity.

Two days a week should be focused on strength and resistance training to help maintain and grow muscle mass and strength. Pick exercises that work all the major muscle groups, such as the legs, hips, abdominals, chest, shoulders, and arms.

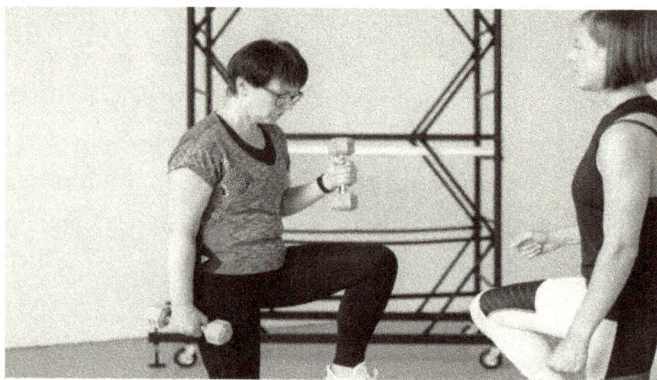

Finally, to improve and work on your balance, you should assign three sessions a week to balance-orientated exercises. Some ideas are to practice standing on one foot, walking backward, or even investing in a wobble board. Again, I have included specific balance-based exercises at the end of each chapter in this book. Yoga inherently also comprises poses that will test and improve your balance as well.

The multicomponent exercise plan listed above can help improve physical function.

Along with a structured exercise program, you should also aim to move more and sit less. Saint-Maurice et al. (2020) looked at the effect of step count on aging, and the results showed that 51% of adults who walked 8000 steps or more had a lower risk of death than those who only took 4000 steps a day. Things like gardening, walking your dog, and just being more aware of your movement can all help increase your step count. Plus, it is free and has wonderful benefits for your mental health as well.

Nutrition

It's been said that food can be medicine, and I agree. What we put into our bodies has a great impact on our wellness. It is certainly a factor we can control when it comes to ensuring longevity.

You should be aiming to eat a well-rounded, balanced diet that contains all the macronutrients, micronutrients, vitamins, and minerals your body needs to function optimally.

Macronutrients are food sources such as protein, carbohydrates, and fats. Your meals should contain all three macronutrients and whole foods that are as fresh as possible.

Some examples of proteins are:

- chicken

- fish

- beef

- steak

- eggs

- shellfish

- deli meat

Some carbohydrate examples are:

- potatoes

- sweet potatoes

- whole grain bread

- legumes

- rice

- whole grain pasta

- squash

- fruits

- various other vegetables

Some healthy fat sources are:

- avocado

- olive oil

- olives

- nuts

- seeds

- grass-fed butter

- ghee

- coconut oil

- avocado oil

- sesame oil

- nut butter

It is not too late to make changes to your current eating habits. Start small and integrate easy routines into your life, such as eating at least one serving of protein at every meal or adding more vegetables to your plate.

Along with healthy eating, it is also important to stay adequately hydrated by drinking enough water daily.

Chat with your healthcare provider if you have any dietary questions or specific requirements.

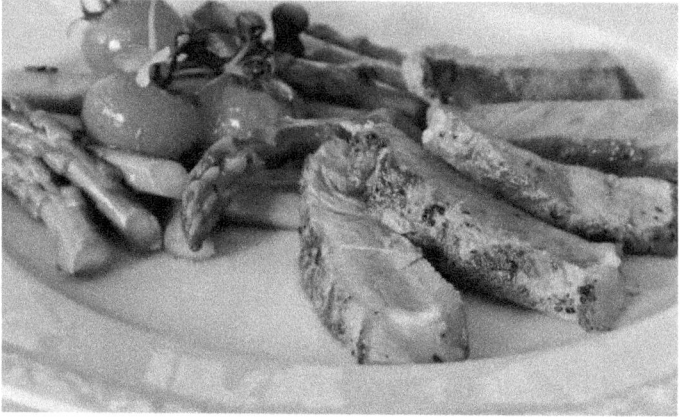

Sleep Routine and Hygiene

Sleep is vital to recovery and well-being. A poor night's sleep can lead to irritability, low mood, forgetfulness, clumsiness, impaired problem-solving abilities, decreased concentration, and even overeating. Studies have shown that a lack of sleep can increase your risk of dementia and worsen depression.

As we age, our need for sleep changes. According to the Centers for Disease Control and Prevention (2019), we need about seven to nine hours of sleep every night.

Try to establish good sleep hygiene and create a sleep routine. Keep to a regular sleep schedule by falling asleep and waking up at the same time each night. You should avoid napping too late in the day, try meditation, and exercise early in the day.

Set up your bedroom so that it is conducive to good sleep. You can invest in some blackout curtains and control the temperature. Remove electronic devices from your room and stop looking at screens for a couple of hours before bed. It is also a good idea to stop drinking and eating a couple of hours before bed (Centers for Disease Control and Prevention, 2019).

Smoking

Regardless of your age or current health, quitting smoking will only benefit you. There is absolutely no benefit to smoking, and the sooner you stop, the quicker you will reap the benefits. It is worth highlighting that the benefits occur immediately as soon as you put out your cigarette.

Studies, which were conducted on approximately 200,000 people, showed that those who quit smoking between the ages of 45 and 54 lived six years longer, and those who quit between 55 to 64 lived about four years longer (Jha et al., 2013).

Your risk of cancer, heart attack, lung disease, and stroke lowers when you quit. Your blood circulation will immediately improve, your sense of taste and smell will increase, and your ability to exercise will become easier.

If you are a smoker, there is no reason to wait.

Alcohol

It has been shown that the use of alcohol has been linked to premature aging, which includes aging of the brain (Sullivan & Pfefferbaum, 2019). Additionally, in an alternative study by Britton et al. (2016), evidence shows that it also has detrimental effects on the health of your heart.

We should be limiting alcohol as well as other substances that potentially cause addiction or reliance. Current guidelines recommend that men stick to two drinks a day and women should only drink one, but there are also certain instances where you should refrain from drinking in its entirety (Rethinking Drinking, n.d.).

Healthcare Management

You must stay abreast of your health by visiting your healthcare provider regularly. This preventative care can help your doctor identify any chronic diseases you may develop earlier on and lessen the risk factors of developing any other diseases, such as cholesterol or high blood pressure.

It is very worthwhile to schedule your doctor's visits at least once a year as a minimum. With the advances in certain testing, equipment, and general medical tools, these visits can improve your health outcomes as you get older.

Ways Around Aging by Taking Care of Our Minds

Along with taking care of our physical health, it is equally as important to invest in our mental health as well. Our mental capacity affects those around us and impacts our relationships, actions, feelings, and moods,

We must learn how to manage the feelings of loneliness, isolation, stress, depression, and other mental health problems that may arise from circumstances related to aging.

Isolation and Loneliness

Isolation is the loss of connection with others, and it occurs when we do not have social contacts and people we can interact with often. On the other hand, loneliness is a feeling—a feeling of being alone or separate from others.

As we get older, we may find ourselves less involved in social activities. This happens for several reasons, either physical or otherwise. We may have lost friends and family members, or we may have trouble getting around and our independence has been hindered. Things like hearing loss, eyesight loss, and general ill health can also make sustaining social connections difficult.

These mental difficulties can affect you physically. The National Institute on Aging (2019) shows that, physically, you may be more susceptible to experience a decline in mental faculty, an increase in depression, and an increased risk of heart complications.

Humans are social creatures. We thrive in communities and are hardwired to need social interaction. Making new social contacts and maintaining our existing social circles can help us feel young (Cornwell & Laumann, 2015).

Positive social interaction brings about feelings of well-being and happiness. We are given a sense of hopefulness and a sense of purpose and community. These interactions greatly improve our quality of life.

It can be as simple as regular phone calls, occasional coffee or dinner meetings, or even taking up a hobby or class and meeting new people.

Stress

Along with sleep, I feel that stress is often overlooked in the wellness space as a significant factor when it comes to aging well. It has been well-established that stress causes changes in the brain. The interesting thing is that it does not matter if the stress is good or bad—the effect of stress is the same.

Memory loss and an increased risk of cognitive diseases are two possible ailments that may occur if we are too stressed (McEwen, 2017).

The stress hormone is known as cortisol, and as we age, our cortisol rates increase. This hormone triggers the changes within the brain, so it is beneficial for us to try to lower our stress and manage our responses to it. Anxiety and stress have been shown to reduce life spans, and data shows that in some cases those who managed their stress levels and emotional stability effectively lived about three years longer than those who didn't (Moffat et al., 2019).

Exercise, social activities, and meditation are some of the tools that you can use to manage your stress levels.

Depression

Low mood and depression can be difficult to pinpoint. It is often believed that sadness is the main determinant of depression, and many use this as a sign that something may be amiss. This is not always the case. Depression can manifest itself in other ways, such as being uninterested in activities, feeling numb, not wanting to engage and discuss feelings with others, as well as being withdrawn. You may also have trouble sleeping and eating.

Depression and extremely low moods affect us physically, and numerous studies have shown that there is a link between depression, metabolic diseases, and cardiovascular diseases (Carney & Freedland, 2016).

As we age, it may become more common to experience mood changes as we navigate this next chapter of our lives, both mentally and physically. I find it rather beneficial to look within and evaluate my thoughts about aging and what it may mean for me.

I aim to see it less as something negative but as another exciting chapter on this life journey. As I hope to show in this book, we can manage the aging process and make it a beautiful and interesting process. There are even studies that will back me up on this! Having a negative attitude toward aging can result in a greater risk of developing negative health outcomes, whilst being more positive can reduce the risk of dementia and obesity (Pietrzak et al., 2016).

There are many treatment options for depression, and you must consult with your health care provider should you experience any symptoms.

Social Enjoyment

As we get older, we need to continue to partake in the activities that we love as well as look for new ones to keep our interest and engagement with others high. They keep our minds active and can stave away mental health diseases.

Myths Around Aging

Let's look at some of the common misconceptions about what it means to get older. We are very aware of the narrative that society has created around getting older, and while there is truth in some of these notions, there are also instances where these ideas are not set in stone and are very nuanced.

You have heard the saying that age is just a number, and it is. As I keep reiterating, we do not need to resign ourselves to a bleak future where our quality of life declines as we play out the remaining chapters of our lives. We get to write the story.

Cognitive Development Declines

It is a common misconception that as we age, our ability to learn new things and rewire neural pathways discontinues and we see a decline in our ability to perform certain cognitive tasks.

We can keep ahead of this by continuing to challenge our minds, and this means continuing to expose ourselves to new tasks and mental stimuli.

According to Anderson (2020), we can develop a *cognitive reserve* that can compensate for any decline that may occur as we age. We can build this by simply taking in a new hobby, learning a language, or even gardening. Here's an idea: Begin yoga!

The most recent studies have also pointed to mindfulness as a cognitive tool that may help preserve mental function. The research, although in its early stages, shows to be very promising.

Driving May Get Difficult

Things such as slower response times, hearing loss, and vision impairment, as well as reduced strength and mobility can affect your driving abilities. But these factors are not tied to a specific age.

I believe that we need to look less at age as the determining factor as to whether or not driving is a safe endeavor and more at the capabilities of each individual to continue to drive safely.

Memory Will Decline

Dementia, Alzheimer's, and other memory-related disorders are fears that we hold in the back of our minds as we get older. And while some mild memory loss and bouts of forgetfulness can occur, please do not dwell on these isolated instances as signs that your memory is in decline.

Forgetting where you put something or forgetting an appointment is part of the parcel of life. Make sure that you keep your brain active and stimulated by continuing to do things like reading, painting, or even just listening to music. These activities will keep the mind active for years.

There are things like our environmental factors that we can control to help us limit the risk of developing Alzheimer's, which include things we looked at previously, such as physical exercise and nutrition.

Depression May Set In

There is a strong link between the process of getting older and the idea that the majority of us seniors are sitting in isolation and loneliness. Social interactions and circumstances may look different as we get older, but we do have a store of beautiful memories of a life well lived to look back on.

Research by Fiske et al. (2009) showed that the rate of depression is far less prevalent in older adults than in younger adults. That being said, if you do begin to feel the symptoms of depression, chat with a family member or close friend. These feelings of anxiety, isolation, and sadness are not a normal part of growing older and some treatments can help.

Be Wary of Exercise

This is one of my pet peeves when it comes to the misconceptions about exercise and growing older. The idea here is that, as seniors, we need to scale down our movement and activity as we stand a greater chance of getting injured.

Yes, as we age, we are going through physical changes, but exercise is a tool that can help minimize the effects of growing older on both our bodies and minds. Find or continue to do an exercise program that you enjoy. I suggest yoga, of course, and you can incorporate it into your current regime, be it weightlifting, walking, running, or any other form of movement you enjoy.

Inactivity is the main cause of physical decline. By not moving, your physical health suffers, and when your physical health suffers, you tend to move less. It is a harmful cycle.

Osteoporosis Only Affects Women

Osteoporosis is a disease that affects the bones, making them more susceptible to fractures and breaks. A lot of emphasis is placed on osteoporosis as a condition that older women should be wary of, but it is equally as important that men are aware of the disease and how to manage it as they age.

According to the National Institute on Aging (n.d.-c), if you are over 50 years old, you have a one in five chance of getting an osteoporosis-related fracture. This can be avoided by exercising, eating enough calcium, not smoking, reducing your alcohol intake, and getting enough vitamin D.

You Need Less Sleep

Sleep is one of the most important tools we have to stay healthy and live fulfilling lives, and I cannot stress how good sleep habits can impact other areas of our lives.

Research indicates that you should continue to aim for seven to nine hours of sleep a night (National Institute of Aging, n.d.). There are certain things you can do to ensure that you get the sleep you deserve and need, including following a bedtime routine and avoiding napping, keeping to a consistent sleep schedule, avoiding electronics before bedtime, exercising, and limiting alcohol and caffeine intake.

Fitness Inspiration

I am fortunate enough to be surrounded by men and women who make their health and fitness a priority. They remind me every day of the importance of taking an hour or so out of my day to move and work on my fitness.

There is an older gentleman who runs around my neighborhood daily. He must be around 65 years old, and he has never missed a day.

Some women in my yoga class have the most amazing control over their bodies. It is inspiring to watch how strong they are and how well their bodies react to the demands that the different yoga positions expect from them. They have certainly put in the work by being consistent.

Along with these regular people that I come across in daily life, there are a couple of better-known ones that inspire me to keep up my health and fitness.

Diane Keaton, who is in her 70s, attributes walking as the exercise that keeps the spring in her step as she ages. Cher manages to fit in exercise five times a week and still surfs. Naomi Watts and Elizabeth Hurley swear by yoga and pilates.

Regardless of the specific style of exercise, these celebrities know that aging can be handled well by keeping up with their exercise routines, eating healthy, and looking after their mental health.

All in their 50s to 70s, these women and men have managed to craft lifestyles that allow them to continue to live largely unaffected by the aging process and in ways that are healthy and full of vitality.

Aging is not one size fits all, and we will all have different experiences of the process as we go through it in our individualized ways. As you will note, there are three main areas that we need to focus on as we age to create a holistic plan to support us. These are the physiological, physiological, and social areas of our lives.

Taking care of our social, mental, and physical health now will build a foundation from which we can age gracefully and as comfortably as possible. Remember, it is never too late to start.

Chapter 2:

Yoga, a Divine Therapy

Let us begin to look at Yoga. I must warn you that we can only dip our toes into the vast ocean of history and information surrounding this practice. I will do my best to give you a broad overview and understanding of this practice. First, let us clear up some misconceptions about yoga.

Misconceptions

Yoga does not subscribe to a particular religion or dogma. It belongs to no single community or belief system but has always been an inclusive tool to nourish one's inner well-being. It is open to everyone and anyone with the desire to partake in yoga, and they can reap the rewards that it has to offer.

Although in Western culture, it is seen primarily as a physical system for health and fitness, it has a far more ambitious goal. It aims to help us align ourselves with the universe and create harmony between us and nature (Basavaraddi, 2015). The process may begin with the body, but the self, mind, and breath are all important elements of the practice.

When we delve into the *Eight Limbs of Yoga* later on in this chapter, you will be introduced to the other aspects of yoga that exist away from the physical realm of exercise.

So, although we may see it as various postures and asanas that can bring about physical wellness, it is important to realize that it is a way of being and that the physical and exercise aspects of it are only a small part of Yoga in its entirety.

The True Meaning of Yoga

Yoga implies a union and means *to unite*. The reference here is that it unites both mind and body as well as person and universe. The outcome is to attain a sense of spiritual growth where the ego is nullified, and you see reality as it is. When you have reached this place known as *nirvana, mukti, or moksha*, you can consider yourself a *yogi* (Basavaraddi, 2015).

I resonate with Sadhguru (n.d.) description of Yoga as being a type of technology for transformation. He describes it as a process where you get to determine who you are as opposed to merely expressing who you are.

He believes yoga can fundamentally change who we are, and I agree. Physically, mentally, and spiritually—I have witnessed this in my life and the life of others.

History and Origins

Yoga's roots are buried thousands upon thousands of years ago, beginning in India where the deity Shiva was seen as the first yogi or Adiyogi and the first guru.

The story goes that along the banks of the Kanti Sarovar Lake, seven men came to plead with Adiyogi to share his yoga wisdom with them so they could deliver it across the world. He eventually conceded and filled these seven men with his knowledge. They were known as *Saptarishis*. They carried the art of Yoga to various parts of the world, including Asia, The Middle East, Northern Africa, and South America.

Although there are specific nuances in each of the seven different branches of Yoga, there are many remarkable parallels that tie them together as well. The evidence of ancient yoga practice can be found at numerous sites across India and Asia.

It was the Sage Maharshi Patanjali who can be accredited with codifying and systematizing the practice of Yoga. He instigated the practice of documenting the literature, which inspired others to do the same, thus creating a great body of knowledge around the practice. Initially, the art of passing down knowledge was done on a mentor-to-student basis. This one-on-one teaching was the primary way to transmit information before the 20th century when group classes became popular (Yogapedia, 2020).

It was between 500 B.C. and 800 A.D. that Yoga went through its most transformative and developmental period led by the religious teachers Mahavir and Buddha. They developed the concepts of the *Five Great Vows* and the *Eightfold Path*, respectively.

As the years have progressed, various teachers have contributed to the different branches and practices of Yoga. It has swept up the world, with Yoga practices being found in almost every city. The one common thread is its profound contribution to our health and well-being.

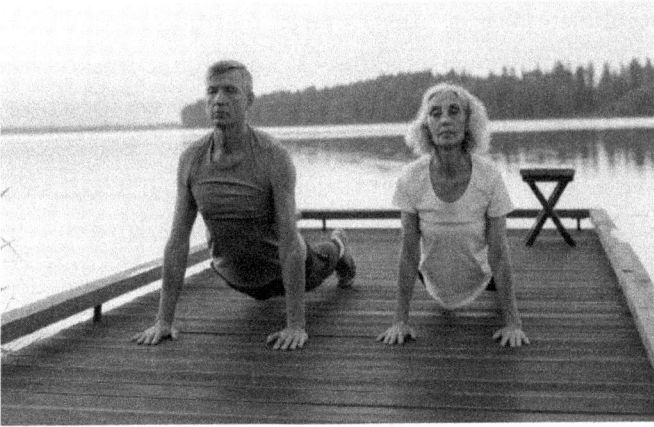

The Four Traditional Paths

Yoga is centered around three distinct parts of our being: our body, mind, emotions, and energy. From here, there are four main paths that each system of yoga falls under.

The four paths are

- Bhakti

- Karma

- Jnana

- Raja

Each person has an individual formula to follow, which is made up of four paths. Because we each have a unique combination, it is often advised that one should work with a guru if one aims to seek Yogi status. Bhakti yoga focuses on our emotions and devotional practices. Karma is associated with action and selfless service. Jnana is tied to our knowledge and self-study—aspects of the mind and intellect. Finally, Raja is related to self-discipline and practice.

In this book, we are concentrating on using yoga as a physical tool to keep us mobile and strong. The other benefits are bonuses that we will also pay attention to. We are well aware of the added benefits of practicing yoga, regardless of the specific form it takes. In this case, to make it as accessible as possible, we are working with chair yoga.

The Eight Limbs of Yoga

As you get more into your yoga practice, you may want to explore the eightfold path of the practice that Buddha was credited with developing.

These eight paths are also known as the *Eight Limbs of Yoga*. These eight paths are instructions for living that will lead the practitioner closer to creating a union between their body, mind, and spirit.

The eight practices are:

1. Yamas

2. Niyamas

3. Asana

4. Pranayama

5. Pratyahara

6. Dharana

7. Dhyana

8. Samadhi

These eight principles focus on creating a practice whereby your actions work toward living a life with more integrity, spirituality, and respect for nature.

Yamas is the five universal, ethical, and moral practices that we should live by which are:

- nonviolence

- truthfulness

- non-stealing

- continence

- non-covetous

Niyamas are five observances:

- contentment

- cleanliness

- spiritual discipline

- study of scriptures

- surrender to God

Asana is associated with physical posture, and Pranayama is with breathing work. Pratyahara focuses on withdrawing the senses, and Dharana focuses on concentration. Finally, Dhyana deals with meditation, and Samadhi with the union with the Divine (Yogapedia, 2020).

The Benefits of Yoga

Yoga is one of the easiest forms of exercise to ease into if you have no prior exercise experience. It is also easy to incorporate into an established exercise routine if you have one already. The benefits are vast and varied, ranging from the physical to the mental. It is a practice that has been around for thousands of years and is well-researched and trusted in its claims of improving health.

Don't just take my word for it though. As you begin your journey, I am positive you will experience most, if not all, of the benefits listed in this section.

Physical Health Benefits of Yoga

From balance to strength, yoga can work wonders on your body as it ages. It can also counteract and alleviate any age-related diseases that may crop up as we get older. Rountree (2022) highlights some of the main benefits of yoga.

Osteoporosis and Osteopenia

We have discussed that as we age, our bone density decreases and we are at greater risk of developing osteopenia or osteoporosis. This can lead to an increased risk of developing fractures if we fall.

Yoga uses your body weight to develop strength and maintain muscle mass. Exercises that use weight and resistance can help keep bones strong and preserve their health. The key here is to focus on poses that physically challenge you, such as lunge poses and balance poses.

This will also help you with your stability and balance and reduce your chance of falling (Rountree, 2022).

If you do have osteopenia or osteoporosis, please chat with your health care provider before beginning your yoga practice. Due to the effect of the disease on the spine, you may need to modify and omit certain poses and movements.

Arthritis

Arthritis, a disease that affects the joints, is a common condition amongst the older population. Characterized by stiff and painful joints, arthritis can limit your range of motion and affect the quality of your everyday life.

Yoga can reduce joint pain and increase flexibility and mobility. Research has also shown that it can reduce inflammation (Rountree, 2022).

Spinal Stenosis

Forward folds and side bend, when executed carefully, can help relieve the pain of spinal stenosis. This is an ailment that can cause pain and numbness in your hips, legs, and, in some instances, your shoulders.

Yoga will not only help alleviate the pain associated with spinal stenosis but also make you more aware of your posture and help you create better posture habits.

Disk and Core Strength

If you have a sore back, you may have disk issues such as herniated, bulging, or slipped disks. Your doctor will be able to diagnose you should this be the case.

Your yoga practice can help as it builds and maintains your core strength. Your core keeps your body and spine strong as well as protected. It consists of your trunk, back, and abdomen. Yoga poses require bracing and stabilization. These poses force your core to stabilize, thus building strength and stability.

Nerve Pain and Neuropathy

Yoga is great for improving blood circulation, and this can help improve the symptoms of nerve pain.

The slow and controlled movements that make up yoga are also great for slowly adjusting your body into a routine where you can control the intensity and movements based on your body's reactions to them.

This body awareness is so important for all aspects of physical health.

Ligaments and Tendons

As we age, so do the ligaments around our joints and muscles. Yoga can help alleviate the wear and tear and stress that we put into our ligaments and make them strong. Tendonitis is the inflammation of the tendons, and tendinopathy is the degradation of the tendons.

If you have ligament issues, yoga will strengthen the muscles around your joints. The muscles will keep the joint protected and allow you to safely continue your daily activity.

The varied movements in yoga will allow you to continue to practice but still avoid working on the area affected by your tendonitis or tendinopathy.

If you already have a ligament injury and are recovering, yoga is adaptable enough to allow you to continue to move and exercise safely.

Muscle Stiffness

As we get older, we produce less collagen, which affects our muscles and myofascial. Collagen helps us remain flexible and supple, but the decline in collagen can lead to inflexibility, stiffness, and imbalance.

Gentle, consistent yoga can help keep you more flexible and can help your general mobility.

Asthma and Breathing Issues

For those who suffer from asthma, yoga is a great way to maintain fitness levels without aggravating your condition. The same principles apply to those who may have additional cardiovascular issues, such as chronic obstructive pulmonary disease (COPD), chronic bronchitis, or emphysema.

Yoga does not elevate the heart rate too much, keeping your breathing calm and controlled. Additionally, the emphasis and focus on the breath can help strengthen our breathing muscles.

Weight Management

Research has shown that consistently practicing yoga can lead to weight reduction. The subjects, aged between 53 and 57, experienced an average of 1.4 kilograms less weight gain than the average adult who did not practice yoga (Kristal et al., 2005).

Manage Type 2 Diabetes and Hypertension

Studies have shown that practicing yoga can have positive effects when managing type 2 diabetes and hypertension.

Studies looked at a group of 30– 50-year-olds who practiced yoga for 40 days and found that there was a dramatic decline in their blood sugar levels (Jain et al., 1993).

Damodaran et al. (2002) determined that yoga could have positive effects on the symptoms associated with hypertension. After three months of consistently practicing yoga daily, subjects saw a decline in blood pressure, cholesterol, blood sugar, and triglycerides.

Mental Health Benefits of Yoga

Reduce Anxiety and Stress

Yoga is known for its relaxation effects, which helps regulate the body's response to stress. When practicing yoga, your heart rate can slow down, your breathing regulates, and your blood pressure lowers (Paturel, 2016).

Research also shows that yoga may aid in producing the hormone gamma-aminobutyric acid (GABA), which has a calming effect on the body (Australian Seniors, 2017).

Boredom and Loneliness

Isolation, loneliness, depression, and lack of social activities and hobbies can hurt your life.

Introducing a new routine can add some excitement to your day and liven up your routine. Adding a new hobby and activity that requires new learning is mentally stimulating as well. Research shows that this helps keep our minds sharp, aiding cognitive function (Australian Seniors, 2017).

Sleep Disruptions and Issues

If you are having trouble winding down and falling asleep, yoga might be just what you need. Controlled and intentional breathing has been proven to bring about states of relaxation. Tapping into this technique can help you fall asleep at the end of the day.

Yoga can also make you physically more tired. Plus, there are specific yoga poses that you can practice at the end of the day to help you fall asleep easier.

Improves Mood

Taking time to focus solely on yourself is an important act of self-care. By partaking in a daily yoga practice, you are giving back to yourself and recognizing that your health and well-being are a priority.

This form of self-care is great to boost your confidence and elevate your mood.

Chair Yoga

What Is Chair Yoga and Who Is It For?

I have already explained what yoga is and where it originated from, so now let's look at what chair yoga is.

Chair yoga is self-explanatory—it is yoga that uses a chair as a prop and has been modified to include all fitness levels regardless of age (Baiera, 2021). It helps decrease the difficulty of yoga and makes it more accessible to a wider population.

Although chair yoga is directed toward the senior population, it can benefit anyone who has mobility issues, such as getting down onto and up off the floor or those who are a falling risk due to eyesight or balance issues. It can help those who experience joint pain or arthritis and will also benefit those who cannot stand for long periods of time or those who may be in a wheelchair.

Chair yoga can be done while seated at work as a quick movement break during the day, and it can also be used by a pregnant woman looking for a gentle form of exercise. Research shows that the benefits are similar to their standing counterparts (Aerobic Activity of Older Adults, n.d.).

As you can tell, chair yoga is a great accessible exercise option for those who cannot handle a strenuous or moderately-strenuous exercise routine. It's perfect for those looking for a gentle workout. And of course, you can always just do chair yoga as a branch of yoga in and of itself.

Not only can anyone practice chair yoga, but it can also be done anywhere. All you need is a couple of poses and a chair. You can do it in an office, boardroom, hotel room, or hospital room—your limits are only bound by your creativity and access to a chair. This makes it a stress-free and accessible exercise habit that can be incorporated into most daily routines. Getting into the habit of exercising regularly is hard enough as it is. The easier the process, the more likely we are to keep up the practice. Chair yoga ticks off all the boxes in that regard.

The Benefits of Chair Yoga

According to Pain Doctor (2019), numerous benefits of chair yoga have been backed up by scientific studies and research.

One such study showed that when senior members participated in two 45-minute chair yoga classes a week over eight weeks, their pain caused by osteoporosis was significantly reduced. The results were that their day-to-day lives significantly improved as the pain was no longer a hindrance to their lifestyles. Additionally, their physical capabilities improved for three months after the study, and they found themselves able to walk faster and with greater ease.

A smaller study investigated the effect that chair yoga had on one's likelihood of falling. The study found the risk was reduced in the participants (Pain Doctor, 2019). Another interesting find was that it also reduced the fear and anxiety that many seniors experienced when it comes to the risk of falling and injuring themselves.

This is just one of the ways that yoga helps to alleviate stress. We are well aware that the art of breathing, which is so central to the practice of yoga, can help promote a relaxed and meditative state, but it is worth mentioning that the movements themselves have the same result.

Exercise in general has positive effects on sleep; chair yoga does as well. It regulates your circadian rhythm, which, in turn, improves your sleep quality.

Taking control of your body and initiating self-care, which you may not have done in several years, can instill a sense of self-confidence and independence. Chair yoga can bring about feelings of accomplishment as you feel your body getting stronger, your physical well-being improving, and your mental health boosting.

Years behind a desk or standing incorrectly can take its toll on our bodies. Chair yoga can improve and maintain your posture, keeping your body functioning optimally and reducing the risk of injuries.

Chair yoga is also affordable and does not require a lot in terms of equipment or training. There is so much information that can be found online, including exercise videos and tutorials. You do not need a gym membership, and you can do it from the comfort of your own home. Remember to reap the benefits and try to be as consistent as possible.

At the end of the day, chair yoga is essentially yoga. The benefits that come with practicing one version can be reaped by practicing the other. They are interchangeable and equally as effective.

Yoga and Your Body

Let's dive into the science around yoga and how and where the different poses work on your body. We will be looking at some of the muscles that the different poses work with to keep you physically strong. Did you know that there are over 600 muscles in our bodies (Spector, 2018)?

Remember, as we age, we lose muscle mass. The muscles in our bodies work in unison to control our bodies and create movements. We must take the necessary actions to maintain and even build as much muscle as we can to keep us strong and functioning optimally (Tangen et al, 2018).

First, we will look at the major muscle groups before looking at more specific groups.

Major Muscle Groups

When muscles contract, they move other body parts. I think it is important for you to have an understanding of the different muscle groups so you know what area of your body you are working on when you exercise. The more you know about yourself physically, the more confident you can be in your routine (Spector, 2018).

The Chest Muscles

The pectorals are the main muscles found in your chest area. These are further divided into parts: the pectoralis major and pectoralis minor.

These muscles help us hold up things in front of our bodies and get to work when we reach for things—they are integral to everyday simple upper-body movements from brushing your hair to putting objects into your pocket.

The Back Muscles

The muscles in your back protect your spinal cord. The back muscles are also the muscles where the movement of your shoulders and neck originate.

The Arm and Shoulder Muscles

The arm and shoulder muscles are made up of the biceps, triceps, and deltoids. The biceps is found in the upper front part of the arm, the triceps in the upper back, and the deltoids are found in the front of the shoulder.

The Abdominal Muscles

The abdominal muscles protect your organs and assist in breathing. Keeping them strong and working optimally can help with your posture.

The muscles on the side of your abdominals are called your obliques. Other muscles that make up your abdominals are the gluteus maximus and medius; the serratus anterior, which is attached to the ribcage; and the psoas major, which helps to flex your hips.

The Legs and Buttock Muscle

Your hamstrings, glutes, quadriceps, and gastrocnemius muscles make up the muscles in your lower body.

Specific Muscle Groups

The Neck

There are four directions that the neck rotates, which are rotation, flexion, extension, and side bending.

The Back

Your back muscles are considered one of the most complex sets of muscles in your body. It begins from your buttocks up to your neck and shoulders. The five muscle groups that can be found here are the latissimus dorsi, rhomboids, trapezius, teres muscle, and erector spinae.

The Shoulders

The shoulder is a joint, but it is specifically a ball and socket joint. The muscle in the shoulder is referred to as the deltoid. The motions of the shoulder are flexion, extension, abduction, adduction, internal rotation, and external rotation. These muscles are responsible for moving your arms upwards.

The Arms

The arm aids the movement of the shoulder. The upper arm muscles help to move the forearm, which consists of everything from the elbow to the hand. The upper arm muscles are known as the bicep and tricep. The bicep is located at the front of your upper arm and the tricep is at the back. Both of these muscles are used when you bend your arms.

The Wrist

The muscles in the wrist help it flex and extend. When you flex, you pull the palm of your hand inward toward your inner wrist, and when you extend, you bend it backward.

The Hands

The hand has an array of muscles that enable it to complete activities that require very fine motor skills. The muscles in the hand are generally very small.

The Abdomen

There are three main muscular regions of the abdomen that all work to stabilize our bodies. These are the rectus abdominis, the transversus abdominis, and the oblique layers. These muscles reinforce our spines and help our trunks to rotate.

The Hips

Like the shoulder, the hip is a ball and socket joint. It is also a weight-bearing joint that can carry quite a significant load. By flexing or extending our hips, we can manipulate the movement of our legs.

The Thigh and Knee

The flexion and extension of our knees are what enable us to walk. There are many large muscle groups associated with the upper leg, such as the quads and hamstrings. The quads are located at the front of your thigh, and they are used for running and walking. The hamstrings are situated on the back of your legs, and they help the quads as you walk.

The Lower Leg and Foot

The calf muscles make up the lower leg. They aid the movement of the ankle and knee and are pivotal for our locomotion. Our foot muscles are also a part of our lower limbs, and like the hands, it has many small intricate muscles that help stabilize the foot and enable us to walk.

The Importance of Your Breathe

Breath and yoga are intertwined. According to Bernier (2020), there are some basic principles you should adhere to make the most of your practice. Keeping these points in mind and practicing them will result in a successful relaxing session.

Usually, when we exercise, we activate our sympathetic nervous system or SNS. You may be familiar with the phrases *flight or fight*. These are the two states that occur when this system is called into action. It involves a quick response to our environment, high energy, adrenaline, and hyper-awareness. It also stimulates the release of certain hormones, such as the stress hormone, cortisol (Green, 2015).

Yoga has the opposite effect, and while stress stimulus can be beneficial to us in small doses, the long-term effects can be detrimental to our health. Yoga activates the parasympathetic nervous system or PSN, which conserves our energy, lowers stress, reduces our blood pressure, and lifts our mood. This results in relaxation and calmness.

What is the key to obtaining this relaxed and calm state? Your breath. When you are breathing deeply and consciously during yoga, you trigger your PNS. Your poses will become more potent, your mind more focused, and your PNS will strengthen, which will lessen your body's need to utilize your SNS.

Harnessing your breath and breathing correctly is a little more complicated than just breathing in and out and requires a bit more concentrated effort and awareness of breathing patterns.

When you inhale, the front of your body expands and your chest opens up. Your belly will also expand as you inhale.

As you exhale and the air is forced out of your lungs, your body will collapse.

Your breathing changes the shape of your body, and we need to align this movement with the movement we do during yoga. The correct sequence of breath needs to connect to the sequence of the pose. We can hamper the effectiveness of the poses as well as negatively affect the body by breathing incorrectly. Correct breathing not only relaxes your mind but also aids in circulating the oxygen through your muscles while you are performing your poses. Of course, this is of great benefit to your body as well.

Here are a few of guidelines to get you started:

1. Inhale when you perform poses that open the front of your body. The inhalation will support the pose as breathing in expands your ribcage and belly.

2. When you are performing a pose that compresses the body, exhale. The same principle applies to exhalations and certain poses that require you to contract.

3. Hold still when you are required to hold your breath. The technique of holding your breath after an inhalation to prolong its effects is often used. When implemented, you should always

hold still in that particular pose and not move during it.

4. On the other hand, you can move if your pause is required after you have exhaled. Your body is now relaxed and less resistant to movements.

5. Make sure that each breath is deliberate and deep. Your breath should also come easily and not be forced, therefore creating no strain on your body. There should be an easy marriage between your breathing and the pose, and as you become more familiar with the movements and the corresponding breathing techniques, this should become automatic.

Your breath also serves to energize your body, and although we aim for full breaths, we should not overfill our lungs to capacity (Wilson, 2015).

Your breath serves as an important part of your practice, and as you become more experienced, it will become second nature to you, I promise!

This has been quite the journey from the beginning of yoga through to its current state and how it can benefit you. You can look forward to increased flexibility by performing the stretches, bends, and twists; improved muscle strength with poses; and better balance and coordination. Of course, the mental benefits cannot be overlooked either.

Your body is a miraculous organism, and I hope you can appreciate all the work that our muscles do to keep us mobile and moving. This is a very brief introduction to anatomy, but as I stated, this information will give you a good overall picture of how and why you should do the poses you are doing. It is also important to have this knowledge of anatomy so that we can have the language tools to discuss what we are doing during each yoga session and why. It also provides us with the confidence and a base understanding of both the practice and ourselves that will enable us to successfully create yoga flows.

If I focused solely on the origins and development of yoga throughout the years, this book would be based on that topic alone, as there is so much material that I could use and would need to include to make it as comprehensive as I would like. Unfortunately, I cannot do that now, but I hope you have a basic understanding of how yoga came into being along with the general guiding principles of the practice. If it piques your interest, I suggest taking some time to delve deeper into the origins of yoga. It is very interesting and can elevate your exercise.

Now, as we move along, we will be looking at the practicalities of beginning your practice. The fun part will now begin.

Chapter 3:

Making Necessary Preparations

Before you begin any exercise routine, please talk to your doctor or health care providers so they can give you the go ahead to proceed. Pay attention to how your body feels and stop if there is any discomfort or pain. If there is anything you may be concerned about, then please, talk to your doctor.

When to Talk to Your Doctor

You should always consult your doctor before you embark on any new exercise plan, whether you are returning to exercise or as a beginner. The Mayo Clinic Staff (2019) has some guidelines that you should follow when embarking on your new exercise routine.

They recommend that you should consult your doctor if you have:

- heart disease

- diabetes

- kidney disease

- cancer or being treated for cancer

- high blood pressure

Some symptoms might be related to heart, lung, or other serious diseases, and if you experience any of these following symptoms, you should consult your doctor:

- Discomfort or pain in your neck, jaw, or arms. This can occur when resting or working out.

- Dizziness or light-headedness while exercising or if you faint during exercise.

- Shortness of breath.

- Swelling of your ankles.

- Elevated heart rate.

- Lower leg pain that goes away when you are at rest.

A good rule of thumb is if you have any doubts or questions, speak to your health care team.

The National Institute on Aging (2020) has compiled a list of questions that you can ask your doctor to determine how to proceed should you require further guidance. Ask your doctor what exercise they may recommend for you in addition to chair yoga. They will have an idea of your medical history and current level of fitness and will recommend something safe for you to do, be it running, weight training, or anything else you may enjoy.

On the other hand, it may also be beneficial to find out what exercise you should be avoiding based on your medical history and fitness levels. If there are certain health ailments that you have, your doctor can also advise how to move forward and develop a plan that enables you to work around these limitations and get you moving again. For example, if you are diabetic, your doctor can advise you on how to plan your meals around exercise as well as adjust your medication.

One of the many benefits of chair yoga (and yoga in general) is that it is a very precise, slow, and mindful exercise. The idea behind it is that you create a very strong mind/body connection. This means you are always in control and aware of how your body is moving and reacting to certain poses and can easily determine if you are comfortable or in pain.

Pay attention and be aware of these feelings when you begin and get an idea of the movements you should be doing more of, less of, or modifying. Remember, as you progress and get more comfortable with the movements, you can begin to make your practice more difficult and increase the intensity. It may seem frustrating at first as you have already adapted yoga by adding in the chair as a prop but trust me, slow and steady is the best path to take in this instance.

The inherent risk is falling. Falls are one of the major causes of injury in the older population, and precautions must be taken to cover this aspect of the practice. You should feel as comfortable in a chair as you do standing up or sitting on a yoga mat (Martins, n.d.). Be aware of any feelings of dizziness.

I see some common ailments that affect my students, including things like osteoporosis, spinal conditions such as degenerative disk disease, inner ear problems, and vertigo. I also have students who have had knee or hip replacement surgery, but with safety precautions in place and clever modification, they all reap the benefits of chair yoga safely.

Make sure that you have a suitable chair placed on a nonslip surface, such as a yoga mat, and if you are in a wheelchair, ensure it is locked in place before you begin. We will go into more detail about equipment as the chapter progresses.

If You Have Diabetes

According to Bell et al. (n.d.), the following precautions should be taken before embarking on a chair yoga session.

Firstly, you should check your blood sugar levels 30–40 minutes before you exercise. If the reading is lower than 200 mg/dL, then you should eat a snack that consists of 15-20 grams of carbohydrates. If it is between 200-300 mg/dL, you do not need to eat anything. If it is 300 mg/dL, then you should refrain from working out and hydrate.

If You Have High Blood Pressure

The most important thing you need to do is take your medication as your doctor has prescribed it and, if possible, take your blood pressure before exercising.

If your systolic reading is 140 or higher and/or your diastolic reading is 100 or higher, you have the following options: avoid weight-bearing exercises and go for a walk or easy cycle and then retake your reading.

When you have high blood pressure, it is recommended that you do not do inversions and stay clear of movements that require excessive twisting or bending.

You should also move between transitions of movements gradually and not rush the practice. This can help reduce dizziness (Martins, 2022).

Getting Started

Once you have been given the go ahead to begin exercising, there are certain things to take into consideration. Make sure that you ease into things slowly, even if you are experienced with exercising. We want to make sure that we give our bodies some time to adjust to the new movements.

Not only can over-exercising lead to injury, but it can also lead to quitting. We will be working on new muscle groups, and the movements may be unfamiliar so we could feel stiff and a bit sore the next day. You do not want to create an unpleasant experience for yourself (National Institute on Aging, n.d.-b).

Along with the workout itself, there are two other elements to a workout routine that are equally as important. These two overlooked elements are warming up and cooling down. You should always ensure that your body is primed for the movement that it is about to do. Warms ups prevent injury and also prepare your muscles to work, which then makes them more efficient and your workout more effective.

Make sure to pay attention to your breathing as deep breaths help you and your joints relax. When practicing chair yoga, be mindful of your posture and keep yourself upright with your feet flat on the floor and your knees aligned over your ankles. You should also avoid straining, bouncing, or jerking movements (Division of Agriculture, n.d.). You should also have water on hand so you can stay hydrated.

I also believe that it is important to set some health and wellness goals for yourself. These do not need to be grandiose but can be something as simple as setting a target for doing two chair yoga sessions a week. Once you have established your short-term goals, you can work on bigger long-term goals. This could be something like being flexible enough to touch your toes with straight legs.

Set your goals and then plan your exercise sessions with yourself. Mark them in your calendar or make a note in your journal. This is your appointment with yourself. You can also recruit a friend or family member to be an accountability partner to help you reach your goals and develop consistency.

Finally, make sure that you track your progress and tweak and change your exercise program as needed. Seeing results and keeping things fresh and exciting will help keep you motivated.

Equipment

One of the great benefits of yoga and chair yoga is that you do not require any special equipment or any large costs involved in practicing. Senior Lifestyle (2020) suggests that you have an armless chair. This should be very stable to prevent any injury.

Should you wish to invest in a chair for your practice, you can find many great ones online. A yoga chair can offer you more support and enable you to do more poses and movements.

Look for features such as lumbar and back support. You can also purchase chairs that have breathable, skin-friendly covers, which are also water, dirt, and dust resistant. Some chairs can be dismantled or folded, so they do not take up a lot of room when you're not using them.

The chair should be placed on a level surface that is not slippery, and you should have enough space to extend your arms and legs and move freely without bumping into anything. If you can, get a chair that has nonslip and non-marking feet.

Wear whatever clothing feels the most comfortable to you, but ideally, it should be clothing that cannot get caught in the chair. Your clothing shouldn't be too restrictive or too baggy and should be breathable to stop you from getting too hot. Your shoes should have a good sole and grip so you do not slip.

When starting, you should also be in the presence of an instructor or friend to ensure safety.

Clothing

You can wear whatever clothing is the most comfortable for you to move in, but here are some common pieces of attire that you can invest in. When you look and feel good, you will move well too.

Yoga Pants

Yoga pants are tight-fitting pants that you can get in a variety of colors and prints. Good quality pants will last you years and are very comfortable to move in.

Loose Pants

If, like me, you prefer looser clothing, you can get a pair of loose pants to wear while you practice. A good option would be a pair of joggers or harem-style pants. The benefit of these loose pants is that, while they allow more room to move, they also have an elastic around the ankle that keeps them in place when you move.

Shorts

If long pants make you too warm when working out, you could wear a pair of shorts. Be aware that some poses require you to be in positions that may leave you exposed if your pants are too loose. Find a pair of shorts that are form-fitting or have a connected interior section to keep you modest!

Tops

Find a top that is form-fitting so it doesn't fall into your face when you do bends. Try to find tops made of breathable material to keep you cool and the sweat at bay.

Sports Bras

Sports bras will offer support even though this is not a high-impact activity. A good sports bra will make the activity more comfortable.

Hair Bands

There is nothing more irritating than having to move your hair out of your eyes and face. Secure your hair with a hair tie or band before you begin your practice.

Yoga Socks

You can either do yoga barefoot, with shoes, or with yoga socks. Unlike regular ones, yoga socks have grips on the bottom so you do not slip.

These are not essential to creating an ideal practice, and as a beginner, you do not need to spring for all these accessories. Simple, everyday comfortable clothing that you already own will be sufficient.

If you are attending a Bikram yoga class, which is heated yoga, it is advisable that you wear very light clothing to counteract the heat. Shorts and shirts are advised, and ideally, they should be made from synthetic, moisture-wicking materials.

Because of the heat, it is best to avoid leggings and large baggy clothing. They will just absorb the sweat and stick to your body. It is also a good idea to bring an extra change of clothes if you would like to shower afterward and freshen up. You will be sweating!

Yoga Etiquette

Yoga for Harmony and Peace (2020) has a couple of guidelines that you can use to ensure that you get the most out of your practice while still adhering to the etiquette and rules that make up a respectful yoga session.

Cleanliness is a core principle of yoga and is referred to as *Śauca*, which is not only regarding the cleanliness of your surroundings and environment but also that of your body and mind.

Most asanas are performed while fasting unless you have a medical condition that requires you to eat before practicing. You should also empty your bladder and bowels before you exercise.

Practice usually begins with a prayer, which signals to our minds that we should be relaxing and easing into our practice. This sets an environment where movement is deliberate, slow, and controlled. Our minds are quiet, and our bodies will follow. The asanas are completed slowly, and we progress to more complicated movements when we are skilled in the basics.

Unless you are instructed otherwise, you will be breathing through your nostrils, and you should not hold your breath. Please refer to the previous sections that cover breathing for more detailed information as this is an important part of your practice.

Just like the start of your practice where you initiated a prayer to quell your mind, the end of practice will culminate in meditation or silence, which gives you time to reflect on your time spent.

Yoga does have some ethical guidelines, which are laid out at the beginning of the *Eight Limbs of Yoga: Yamas and Niyamas*. You can refer back to the previous sections that highlight the specific observances they require.

There are a couple of things you should be conscious of and refrain from doing when practicing yoga.

The first is that you should always practice in a well-rested and energized state of mind. Your practice should not be done in a hurry when you are exhausted or anxious.

Refrain from eating about two to three hours before your practice and wait 30 minutes afterward, and do not follow your yoga practice with a strenuous bout of exercise.

We have taken a lovely route to tell the story of yoga from its beginnings and origins, its effects on the body and breathing, to the equipment and attire we should wear as we practice. We are up to date and where we need to be as we head into the next section of the book. We will start with the warm-ups and then work our way through the various programs from low intensity to high intensity. You will find a program that suits you and your fitness levels.

Chapter 4:

Take a Moment... and Warm Up!

I understand you are eager to get going and warming up can seem like a chore. We must make sure that we are ready to exercise and our joints and muscles are primed for the movements we will be asking them to perform.

Regardless of how relaxed or moderate your particular session may be, it is still very important to warm up properly. Let's go through some of the reasons why and then how.

Why Is Warming up so Important?

Warming up increases your blood flow and gets it moving to all parts of the body efficiently, especially your muscles. Your breathing will become elevated as well as your heart rate, and different energy reactions in your body will be triggered (Fitnessfit, n.d.).

Warming up allows your body to comfortably adapt to the above changes that occur, so it does not become a shock to your system.

By forgoing your warm-up, you may also hamper your recovery as well as put yourself at greater risk for sore muscles and fatigue. You may even have a less effective workout than if you had warmed up as your body will not be functioning at its optimal levels.

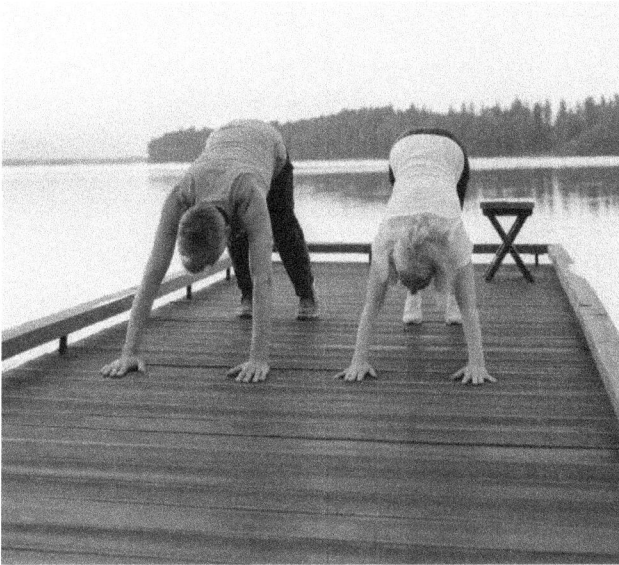

Harvard Health Publishing (2020) suggests that a simple five-to-ten-minute warm-up will be sufficient, and each warm-up will look different depending on the movements you may be doing that day.

Usually, most warm-ups will begin by raising your heart rate using a form of cardio. This could be doing jumping jacks, going on a brisk walk, or even marching on the spot. You will also be working out your whole body as opposed to just your upper or lower sections, so your warm-up will be full-body focused.

If there are sections of your body that feel a little tighter or stiff, spend more time warming up that area and priming it for your practice. Use dynamic stretching as opposed to static as it benefits the joints and muscles more but keep the intensity low—you do not want to tire yourself out before you get to the yoga practice itself (Tomko, 2020).

I have a simple strategy that covers most of my bases when it comes to warming up. One of the first things I do is foam roll or pain ball my sore muscles. A foam roller is a device that enables you to perform a self-massage. Foam rolling can help get rid of knots, tension, or trigger points that may hinder your practice. Once I have foam rolled, I will get my heart rate up. I usually alternate between some easy skipping and jumping jacks. If the weather is good, I will take a brisk walk around the neighborhood.

Secondly, I incorporate any corrective exercises into my warm-up. These are exercises that I have been given to work on. One is to stand on one leg for as long as I can manage as a means to work on my balance. This serves as a way to get me to do the boring exercises prescribed to me and warm-up at the same time with different types of movements.

Finally, as part of my warm-up, I also work on my mobility and flexibility. After activating my muscles with simple activation drills, I will work on my mobility by putting my joints through their full range of motion and prepping them for the yoga session.

Common Warm-up Movements

There are a variety of warm-up movements that you can include at the beginning of any chair yoga routine. These movements are selected to increase the range of motion of your spine and to warm up your torso muscles. They focus on your upper and middle back as well as your psoas.

Hand Clenches

1. Begin by sitting upright in your chair with your feet planted firmly on the ground.

2. Place your palms on each of your thighs.

3. Keep your gaze forward and your spine elongated.

4. Inhale and raise your arms out in front of you, palms facing downwards.

5. Open your hands and stretch your fingers out wide. Hold for a count of five.

6. Clench your fists tightly. Hold for a count of five.

7. Repeat for 20 repetitions.

Ankle Crank on Chair

1. Begin by sitting upright in your chair with your feet planted firmly on the ground.

2. Place your palms on each of your thighs.

3. Keep your gaze forward and your spine elongated.

4. Inhale and bring your right foot to rest on your left knee. Your foot should be hanging loose on the other side of your leg.

5. Inhale and begin to rotate your ankle clockwise for 10 repetitions.

6. Next, rotate your ankle anti clockwise for 10 repetitions.

7. Return to the starting position.

8. Inhale and bring your left foot to rest on your right knee. Your foot should be hanging loose on the other side of your leg.

9. Inhale and begin to rotate your ankle anticlockwise for 10 repetitions.

10. Next, rotate your ankle in a clockwise direction for 10 repetitions.

11. Return to the starting position.

Sun Breathes on Chair

1. Begin by sitting upright in your chair with your feet planted firmly on the ground.

2. Place your palms on each of your thighs.

3. Keep your gaze forward and your spine elongated.

4. Inhale and bring your palms to your heart's center and pause.

5. Exhale and bring your arms outward to your side.

6. Move slowly and with intention.

7. Finish your exhale by bringing your palms back to the top of your thighs.

Chair Neck Rolls

1. Begin by sitting upright in your chair with your feet planted firmly on the ground.

2. Place your palms on each of your thighs.

3. Keep your gaze forward and your spine elongated.

4. Exhale as you move your right ear toward your right shoulder.

5. On your inhale, return your head to the middle starting position.

6. Exhale as you move your left ear toward your right shoulder.

7. On your inhale, return your head to the middle starting position.

Chair Upward Hand Stretch

1. Begin by sitting upright in your chair with your feet planted firmly on the ground.

2. Place your palms on each of your thighs.

3. Keep your gaze forward and your spine elongated.

4. Raise your arms out in front of you and interlock them.

5. Stretch them out and remain in this position for two to three breaths.

6. Inhale and raise your arms above your head, keeping them interlocked.

7. Hold them above the crown of your head and stretch them upward. Exhale.

8. Remain here for five to six breaths.

9. With each breath, deepen your stretch.

10. Relax and lower to the starting position.

Chair Seated Shoulder Circles

1. Begin by sitting upright in your chair with your feet planted firmly on the ground.

2. Place your palms on each of your thighs.

3. Keep your gaze forward and your spine elongated.

4. With your elbows pointing outwards, bring the tips of your fingers to rest on your shoulders.

5. Leading with your elbows, move your arms forward in a circular motion. Repeat for the desired amount of revolutions.

6. Leading with your elbows, move your arms backward in a circular motion. Repeat for the desired amount of revolutions.

Chair Seated Side Stretch

1. Begin by sitting upright in your chair with your feet planted firmly on the ground.

2. Place your palms on each of your thighs.

3. Keep your gaze forward and your spine elongated.

4. Inhale and raise your right arm toward the ceiling extending over your head to the left side as far as you can go.

5. Gently tilt your chin and neck toward the left.

6. Exhale completely and stay in that position. Take three more breaths.

7. Inhale while extending your right arm and lowering it back to your lap.

8. While you relax your shoulders and upper back, exhale.

9. Inhale and raise your left arm toward the ceiling extending it over your head to the right side as far as you can.

10. Gently tilt your chin and neck toward the right.

11. Exhale completely and stay in that position. Take three more breaths.

12. Inhale while extending your left arm and lowering it back to your lap.

13. While you relax your shoulders and upper back, exhale.

Chair Torso Circles

1. Begin by sitting upright in your chair with your feet planted firmly on the ground.

2. Place your palms on each of your thighs.

3. Keep your gaze forward and your spine elongated.

4. Place your hands on your hips.

5. Rotate your torso by pushing your chest forward and moving it in a counterclockwise direction.

6. Return to the center.

7. Repeat in the other direction.

Single Arm and Alternating Leg Raise

1. Begin by sitting upright in your chair with your feet planted firmly on the ground.

2. Place your palms on each of your thighs.

3. Keep your gaze forward and your spine elongated.

4. Inhale and lift your left arm straight above you in line with your ear.

5. As you raise your left arm, raise the right leg and straighten it out in front of you.

6. Exhale and lower both limbs to the starting position.

7. Inhale and lift your right arm straight above you in line with your ear.

8. As you raise your right arm, raise the left leg and straighten it out in front of you.

9. Exhale and lower both limbs to the starting position.

Chair Flexing Foot Pose

1. Begin by sitting upright in your chair with your feet planted firmly on the ground.

2. Place your palms on each of your thighs.

3. Keep your gaze forward and your spine elongated.

4. Inhale as you raise your left leg to an approximately 40° angle. Keep your right leg flat on the ground.

5. Hold in position and flex your foot toward your shin, and then flex your foot toward your heel.

6. Return your leg to the floor.

7. Inhale as you raise your right leg to an approximately 40° angle. Keep your left leg flat on the ground.

8. Hold in position and flex your foot toward your shin, and then flex your foot toward your heel.

9. Return your leg to the floor.

Seated Marches

1. Begin by sitting upright in your chair with your feet planted firmly on the ground.

2. Place your arms at your side.

3. Keep your gaze forward and your spine elongated.

4. Inhale as you bring your left thigh as high up as you can, keeping your leg bent.

5. Exhale as you return to the starting position.

6. Inhale as you bring your right thigh as high up as you can, keeping your leg bent.

7. Exhale as you return to the starting position.

8. Repeat for 20 marches.

Seated Shoulder Circles

This movement targets your arms and shoulders.

1. Begin by sitting upright in your chair with your feet planted firmly on the ground.

2. Place your arms at your side.

3. Keep your gaze forward and your spine elongated.

4. Inhale and bring your fingertips to rest on your shoulders, your elbows pointed away from your body to the side.

5. Rotate your elbow and shoulders forward. Begin with small circles and gradually progress to bigger ones.

6. Rotate 20 times forward.

7. Pause and rotate 20 times backward.

Seated Pillow Squeezes

1. Begin by sitting upright in your chair with your feet planted firmly on the ground.

2. Place your arms at your side.

3. Keep your gaze forward and your spine elongated.

4. Put a pillow between your thighs and knees.

5. Focus on contracting your inner thigh muscles and squeezing the pillow.

6. Hold the squeeze for three seconds.

7. Relax.

8. Repeat 12 times.

Seated Clamshells

1. Begin by sitting upright in your chair with your feet planted firmly on the ground.

2. Place your palms on the outside of each of your thighs just above the knee. Your hands will provide resistance to this movement.

3. Keep your gaze forward and your spine elongated.

4. Inhale, and as you exhale, move your knees toward your hands. Contract the muscles on the outside of your hips as you do so. Your hands are creating the resistance, and you can create the force and effort required.

5. Hold for three seconds and then relax.

6. Repeat 12 times

Seated Knee Extensions

1. Begin by sitting upright in your chair with your feet planted firmly on the ground.

2. Place your palms on each of your thighs.

3. Keep your gaze forward and your spine elongated.

4. Take a big inhale, and as you exhale, bend your left knee before extending and straightening it out in front of you.

5. Focus on squeezing your quadricep, which is the big muscle at the front of your thigh.

6. Hold this position for three seconds. Return to the starting position.

7. Take a big inhale, and as you exhale, bend your right knee before extending and straightening it out in front of you.

8. Focus on squeezing your quadricep, which is the big muscle at the front of your thigh.

9. Perform this for 15 repetitions on each side or alternate legs and perform 30 repetitions in total.

Ankle Pumps With Straight Knees

1. Begin by sitting upright in your chair with your feet planted firmly on the ground.

2. Place your palms on each of your thighs.

3. Keep your gaze forward and your spine elongated.

4. Straighten your legs out in front of you, keeping your knees straight.*

5. Flex your foot downwards toward the floor.

6. Hold for three seconds.

7. Flex your foot upwards toward the ceiling.

8. Hold for three seconds.

9. Repeat 1o times.

*If it is too difficult to hold both legs elevated at the same time, you can do each leg individually and alternate the exercise.

Warm-up Routine

Before we get started, let's bear in mind and remember that we should always be very aware of our breath while moving through these poses. This will set the tone for the rest of the practice.

Cardio Warm-up Options

First, we will get our heart rate elevated before we take to the chair and prepare for our practice. We took some inspiration from Freytag (2022) and Kamb (2023) when we were putting together ideas for easy cardio movements.

You can do any form of cardio to elevate your heart rate, so pick one of the below options that you're comfortable with:

- Thirty seconds to one minute of walking jacks, or if you are comfortable, jumping jacks.

- Ten repetitions of forward leg swings and ten repetitions of side leg swings on each leg.

- Thirty seconds to one minute of marching on the spot while swinging your arms.

- Thirty seconds of light jogging on the spot.

- Thirty seconds to one minute of swinging toe touches.

- Thirty seconds of jumping rope.

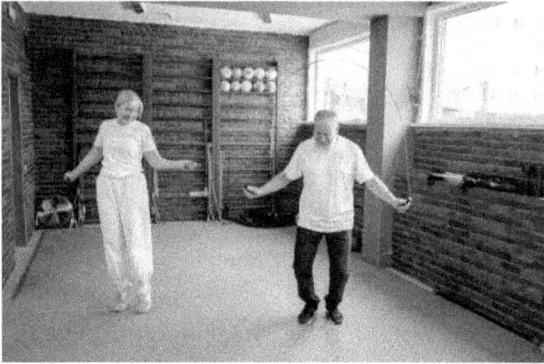

Chair Based on Warm-up

1. Begin by sitting upright in your chair with your feet planted firmly on the ground.

2. Place your palms on each of your thighs.

3. Keep your gaze forward and your spine elongated.

4. Take a deep breath through your nose and deep into your belly.

5. Exhale with an audible sigh and repeat two more times.

6. Bring your arms out in front of you with your palms together.

7. As you exhale, stretch out your arms to your side, keeping your palms facing forward. This movement should take four seconds to complete.

8. Repeat five times.

9. Return to your starting position and slowly rock your head from side to side by bringing your left ear to your left shoulder and your right ear to your right shoulder.

10. Repeat 1o times.

11. Return to your starting position.

12. Inhale and raise your left arm over your head.

13. Keep your torso facing forward as you stretch as far as you can go while remaining seated on the chair.

14. Exhale and return to the starting position.

15. Inhale and raise your right arm over your head.

16. Keep your torso facing forward as you stretch as far as you can go while remaining seated on the chair.

17. Repeat 10 times.

18. Exhale and return to the starting position.

19. You should feel a stretch in your ribcage and along the side of your body.

20. Shrug your shoulders upward and rotate them backward and down.

21. Repeat 10 times.

22. Shrug your shoulders upward and rotate them forward and down.

23. Repeat 10 times and return to the starting position.

24. Sit up tall and open your legs wide.

25. Exhale and bend forward, leading with your chest toward your left knee.

26. Inhale and return to your upright position.

27. Exhale and bend forward, leading with your chest toward your right knee.

28. Repeat 10 times.

29. Inhale and return to your upright position.

30. Raise your arms straight in front of you and wiggle every single finger. Do this for 30 seconds.

31. Move your arms out toward the side and continue to do the same for 30 seconds.

32. Move your arms back to the center and stretch your fingers outwards as wide as you can and then ball them tightly into fists.

33. Repeat this 20 times.

34. Move your arms back out to your side, keeping your fists clenched, and rotate your wrists forward 10 times.

35. Rotate backward 10 times.

36. Return to your starting position.

37. Place your hands on your upper thigh and slowly walk them down your legs, going as far down as you feel comfortable but keeping your back flat against the chair.

38. Once you have walked your hands as far down your legs as you can, walk them back up.

39. Repeat five times.

40. Extend your left leg out in front of you with the heel on the ground and your toes pointed toward the ceiling.

41. Inhale and point your toes toward the floor. Exhale and point your toes backward toward your shins.

42. Repeat 10 times.

43. Extend your right leg out in front of you with the heel on the ground and your toes pointed toward the ceiling.

44. Inhale and point your toes toward the floor. Exhale and point your toes backward toward your shins.

45. Repeat 10 times.

46. Extend your left leg out in front of you again, keeping it slightly elevated off the floor. Rotate your ankle in a clockwise direction for 10 revolutions. Inhale and exhale for each circle. Rotate in an anticlockwise direction for 10 revolutions.

47. Return to the starting position.

48. Extend your right leg out in front of you again, keeping it slightly elevated off the floor. Rotate

your ankle in a clockwise direction for 10 revolutions. Inhale and exhale for each circle. Rotate in an anticlockwise direction for 10 revolutions.

49. Return to the starting position.

50. Take a deep breath through your nose and into your belly.

51. Exhale with an audible sigh and repeat two more times.

What About the Cooldown?

Cooling down is just as important as warming up. Cooling down will benefit your body in numerous ways, which we will explore further in this section.

Your cooldown does not need to be too long and take up much of your time. I know you are busy, but you should aim to do one after each session.

The cooldown helps your body return to a relaxed state. According to Purdie (2022), the main purpose of a cooldown is to return the body to the pre-exercise state. The way you approach this can vary. You can go with the physical route, mental route, or combine both of them.

Some ideas are to take a walk or slow jog to bring your heart rate down, or you could stretch. If you prefer, you could even do a short meditation session.

If done properly, a cooldown will help mitigate the effects of delayed onset muscle soreness. This is the term for the pain or stiffness you may feel in your muscles after exercise. This is caused by small tears in your muscles, but the effects of this can be lessened by cooling down properly. When we do some sort of aerobic activity after exercise, such as a light jog, we help blood circulate in the body as well as remove any waste buildup. This helps us recover quicker.

You will also mentally prepare yourself for the nonphysical activity that follows.

If you battle with your flexibility, then I suggest you use your cooldown time to get some stretching exercises in. This is the prime time to do so as your muscles are warm and primed to bend further and move through a full range of motion.

Here is a quick two-step cooldown routine you can incorporate into your sessions:

1. Walk for five minutes and bring your heart rate down to approximately 120 beats per minute.

2. Begin stretching and hold each of your selected stretches for 30 seconds.

Simple, right?

Congratulations, you have taken tangible steps toward changing your health and wellness for the better! The simple act of warming up will become a part of your routine from which your practice will evolve and grow.

Consider this a milestone. The added beauty of the warm-up is that on days when I don't feel like exercising and have no desire to do my chair yoga practice, I convince myself to just do the warm-up. I reason that if I do the warm-up and still do not feel like practicing, then I have given it some effort and can walk away knowing I tried.

The sneaky thing is that hardly happens, and once I have gone through the motions of my warm-up, I am eager to continue. I suggest using this strategy as well. It works!

The rest of the chapters will progress through the different movements and practices that you can do based on the intensity of the exercise you are wanting, capable of, and willing to do. It will range from low, moderate, and higher intensities.

Part Two: Easy-To-Follow Chair Yoga Programs for Seniors

Chapter 5:

Low-Intensity Chair Yoga

Program

This exercise is a low-intensity program that is targeted toward those over 70 years of age, but it can be used by anyone looking for a less strenuous workout or has certain limitations.

First, we will do a quick warm-up routine, then you may choose three to five poses for each specific muscle group that we will be focusing on during this session: the upper body, midsection, and lower body.

Warm-up

1. We will begin by marching on the spot for 30–60 seconds. Begin by standing up straight next to your chair; you can use the chair for support.

2. Lift your left leg, keeping your knee bent, and raise it as high as you feel comfortable.

3. Lower to a standing position.

4. Lift your right leg, keeping your knee bent, and raise it as high as you feel comfortable.

5. Repeat for 30–60 seconds.

6. Raise your hands out to the side, palms facing downward.

7. Moving from your shoulder, rotate your arms forward in small circles.

8. Repeat for 30 seconds.

9. Repeat this sequence for three to five minutes (Kristal et al., 2005).

As you put together your program, I would like you to select three to five poses that you will be doing for each muscle group. Be as creative as you like and modify them to your capabilities.

Chair Yoga Upper-Body Exercises

These exercises will target your upper body. The main muscles we will be focusing on are the biceps, triceps, shoulders, forearms, wrists, hands, and upper back. Many of these poses will work to relax your upper back and shoulders as well as build stability in your shoulder joints (Stelter, 2022).

Warrior I (Virabhadrasana I)

This pose will open up your upper body and heal your breathing.

1. Begin by sitting upright in your chair with your feet planted firmly on the ground.

2. Place your arms on either side of you.

3. Keep your gaze forward and your spine elongated.

4. Inhale and lift your arms to your side and raise them over your head to meet palm to palm.

5. Intertwine your fingers but keep your pointer and thumb extended. You will be pointing at the ceiling.

6. Exhale and gently roll your shoulders away from your ears and relax your shoulder blades. You should feel your shoulder blades engage.

7. Breathe for five counts before you return to the starting position.

Eagle Arms

This position opens up and stretches your upper back

and shoulders.

1. Begin by sitting upright in your chair with your feet planted firmly on the ground.

2. Place your arms on either side of you.

3. Keep your gaze forward and your spine elongated.

4. As you inhale, extend your arms out to the side of your body.

5. As you exhale, extend them out in front of you. Place your right arm under your left arm. Grab each shoulder with the opposite hand similar to hugging yourself.

6. Depending on your flexibility, you could continue to wrap your forearms around each other until your right fingers are joined with your left palm.

7. On your inhale, lift your elbows higher.

8. On your exhale, gently relax your shoulders and roll them away from your ears.

9. Hold for five to eight breaths, continuing to lift your elbows and release your shoulders.

Reverse Arm Hold

This is a great position to open up your chest and it can help you should you have breathing difficulties.

1. Begin by sitting slightly forward and upright in your chair with your feet planted firmly on the ground.

2. Place your arms on either side of you.

3. Keep your gaze forward and your spine elongated.

4. Inhale and stretch your arms out to the side of you with your palms facing downward.

5. Exhale and roll both of your shoulders slightly forward. Your palms should now be facing behind you.

6. Bending at the elbows, bring your arms behind your back.

7. Clasp your left hand on your right hand and gently pull them apart, creating resistance. Hold for five slow breaths.

8. Return to the starting position.

9. Repeat, but this time, clasp your right hand on your left hand and gently pull them apart, creating resistance. Hold for five slow breaths.

Overhead Stretch

This movement opens up your chest, back, and shoulders.

1. Begin by sitting upright in your chair with your feet planted firmly on the ground.

2. Place your arms on either side of you.

3. Keep your gaze forward and your spine elongated.

4. Inhale and raise your hands above your head, in line with your ears and palms facing each other.

5. Hold for a breath, and then exhale and lower your arms back to starting position.

6. Repeat eight times.

Neck Stretch

This movement creates flexibility and mobility in your neck and upper spine.

1. Begin by sitting slightly forward and upright in your chair with your feet planted firmly on the ground.

2. Place your arms on either side of you and hold the base of your chair.

3. Keep your gaze forward and your spine elongated.

4. Exhale as you tilt your chin upward toward the ceiling.

5. Keep your right hand grasping the bottom of the chair and bring your left hand up and place it on your left temple.

6. Inhale, and as you exhale, gently move your left ear toward your left shoulder.

7. Take five breaths and return to starting.

8. Keep your left hand grasping the bottom of the chair and bring your right hand up and place it on your left temple.

9. Inhale, and as you exhale, gently move your right ear toward your right shoulder.

10. Take five breaths and return to starting.

Seated Mountain

This pose works the arms, shoulders, wrists, and midline. It is also a great transitionary pose to be used between others.

1. Begin by sitting upright in your chair with your feet planted firmly on the ground. The distance between your legs should be a fist wide and your knees should be directly over your ankles.

2. Place your arms on either side of you.

3. Keep your gaze forward and your spine elongated.

4. Take a deep breath, and as you exhale, shift down into your sit bones (these are the two points of your buttocks that are planted into the seat).

5. Breathe in again, and as you exhale, roll your shoulders backward and down.

6. Pull your belly button toward your spine, activating your core.

7. Continue inhaling and exhaling in this manner for 20 breaths.

Seated Cactus Arms

This pose builds strength in your neck, arms, and shoulders.

1. Begin by sitting upright in your chair with your feet planted firmly on the ground.

2. Place your hands on your thighs.

3. Keep your gaze forward and your spine elongated.

4. Inhale as you bring your arms to shoulder height, keeping them bent at the elbows and your palms facing forward.

5. Exhale and spread your fingers out wide.

6. Hold for 10 breaths.

Seated Palm Tree Pose Side Bend Flow

This flow works your upper body, specifically your biceps, triceps, upper back, and psoas.

1. Begin by sitting upright in your chair with your feet planted firmly on the ground.

2. Place your hands on your thighs.

3. Keep your gaze forward and your spine elongated.

4. Inhale and bring your arms up overhead, keeping them in line with your ears, and interlock your fingers.

5. Exhale and bend your torso to the right and keep your body facing the front.

6. Inhale and return to the center.

7. Exhale and bend your torso to the left, keeping your body facing the front.

8. Inhale and return to the center.

Repeat for 20 alternating repetitions.

Chair Yoga Lower-Body Exercises

These exercises will target your lower body. The main muscles we will be focusing on are the calves, quadriceps. hamstrings, and glutes.

These movements were selected for those of you who may have mobility issues, are recovering from surgery on your lower body, or have balance problems and concerns that inhibit you from being upright while exercising.

Seated External Hip Rotation Pose

This is a lovely pose to open up your hips and work your knees.

1. Begin by sitting upright in your chair with your feet planted firmly on the ground.

2. Place your palms on each of your thighs.

3. Keep your gaze forward and your spine elongated.

4. Inhale and draw your left leg out to the side of your chair, keeping your torso and hips facing forward.

5. Hold for three breaths.

6. Exhale and return to the center.

7. Inhale and draw your right leg out to the side of your chair, keeping your torso and hips facing forward.

8. Hold for three breaths.

9. Return to the center.

Ankle Crank on Chair

This works the feet and ankles.

1. Begin by sitting upright in your chair with your feet planted firmly on the ground.

2. Place your palms on each of your thighs.

3. Keep your gaze forward and your spine elongated.

4. Inhale and bring your right foot to rest on your left knee. Your foot should be hanging loose on the other side of your leg.

5. Inhale and begin to rotate your ankle clockwise for 10 repetitions.

6. After that, rotate your ankle in an anticlockwise direction for 10 repetitions.

7. Return to the starting position.

8. Inhale and bring your left foot to rest on your right knee. Your foot should be hanging loose on the other side of your leg.

9. Inhale and begin to rotate your ankle clockwise for 10 repetitions.

10. After that, rotate your ankle in an anticlockwise direction for 10 repetitions.

11. Return to the starting position.

Single Leg Stretch (Janu Sirsasana)

This pose works the calves, hamstrings, and quads.

1. Begin by sitting slightly forward and upright in your chair with your feet planted firmly on the ground.

2. Place your arms on either side of you and hold the base of your chair.

3. Keep your gaze forward and your spine elongated.

4. Stretch your right leg out in front of you so your leg is straight, your heel is on the floor, and your toes are pointed toward the ceiling. The further forward you are in the chair, the easier it is to straighten out your leg.

5. Place both of your hands on your outstretched leg.

6. Inhale and rise through your spine.

7. Exhale and begin walking your hands down your outstretched leg.

8. Go as far as you feel comfortable, paying attention to how this feels and making sure you do not force or strain anything.

9. Take even inhales and exhales in this position, attempting to go deeper into the position with each breath.

10. After about five breaths, slowly return to the starting position.

11. Repeat on the other leg.

Seated Tree Pose

This pose works the lower body and is often used to improve balance.

1. Begin by sitting upright in your chair with your feet planted firmly on the ground.

2. Place your arms on either side of you.

3. Keep your gaze forward and your spine elongated.

4. Shift your weight onto your left foot and raise your right foot onto your toes.

5. Turn your right knee out to the side, keeping your hips facing forward, your toes and feet on the ground and in contact with each other.

6. Keep your core engaged and raise your arms over your head.

7. Hold for eight breaths.

8. Come back to your starting position.

9. Shift your weight onto your right foot and raise your left foot onto your toes.

10. Turn your left knee out to the side, keeping your hips facing forward, your toes and feet on the ground and in contact with each other.

11. Keep your core engaged and raise your arms over your head.

12. Hold for eight breaths.

13. Come back to your starting position.

Arm and Leg Raise

This pose focuses on the hips and quads.

1. Begin by sitting upright in your chair with your feet planted firmly on the ground.

2. Place your arms on either side of you.

3. Keep your gaze forward and your spine elongated.

4. Inhale and raise your left leg out in front of you while simultaneously raising your right arm in front of you and toward your ear.

5. Hold for five breaths, keeping your midline engaged by pulling your belly button toward your spine.

6. Return to the starting position.

7. Inhale and raise your right leg out in front of you while simultaneously raising your left arm in front of you and toward your ear.

8. Hold for five breaths, keeping your midline engaged by pulling your belly button toward your spine.

9. Return to the starting position.

Chair Pigeon Pose (Eka Pada Rajakapotasana)

This is a great pose for those of you with tight hips and glutes. It also targets the hamstrings and ankles.

1. Begin by sitting slightly forward and upright in your chair with your feet planted firmly on the ground.

2. Place your arms on either side of you.

3. Keep your gaze forward and your spine elongated.

4. Rest your left ankle on the top of your right knee.

5. Inhale, and on your exhale, fold forward from your hips, keeping your back straight.

6. Take five breaths in this position and return to the starting position.

7. Rest your right ankle on the top of your left knee.

8. Inhale, and on your exhale, fold forward from your hips, keeping your back straight.

9. Take five breaths in this pose and return to the starting position.

Chair Forward Bend Pose (Uttanasana)

This pose not only works your hamstrings but also your upper back.

1. Begin by sitting upright in your chair with your

feet planted firmly on the ground. Your knees should be touching.

2. Place your arms on either side of you.

3. Keep your gaze forward and your spine elongated.

4. Take a deep breath in, and on your exhale, slowly bend forward from your hips. You should be moving single vertebrae at a time.

5. Lean as far forward as you can while still maintaining comfort.

6. Let your head rest on your lap with your arms dangling in front of you.

7. Hold this position for five to ten breaths.

8. Inhale and raise yourself up gently, vertebra by vertebrae, ending with your hands up over your head.

9. Repeat five times.

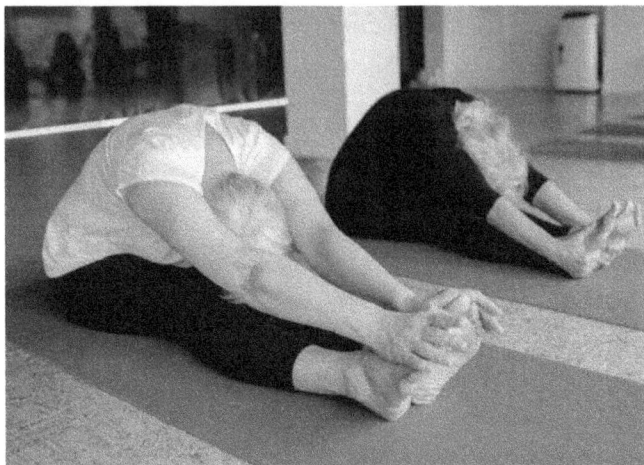

Chair Goddess Pose With Hands and Knees Forward

This pose is very beneficial for your hips.

1. Begin by sitting upright in your chair with your
    feet planted firmly on the ground and your legs
    out wide, your toes pointing outwards and your
    knees over your ankles.

2. Place your arms on your thighs.

3. Keep your gaze forward and your spine
    elongated.

4. Inhale, and on your exhale, lean forward from
    your hips, keeping your torso elongated.

5. Inhale and return to the starting position.

6. Repeat for five to eight repetitions.

Chair Yoga Full-Body Exercises

These exercises will target your torso and midline, which includes your core and lower and upper back. The main muscles we will be focusing on are the abdominal core muscles and back.

Chair Spinal Twist Pose (Ardha Matsyendrasana)

This pose works your spine and encourages flexibility and mobility. It also targets your core muscles.

1. Begin by sitting slightly forward and upright in your chair with your feet planted firmly on the ground.

2. Place your arms on either side of you.

3. Keep your gaze forward and your spine elongated.

4. Inhale as you raise your hands to your side.

5. Gently twist your upper body to your right as you exhale and lower your arms as you do so. Your right hand can gently help you twist by using the

support of the chair. Your left hand will return to your side.

6. Gently look over your right shoulder.

7. Hold the twist for five breaths and release.

8. Repeat on the other side.

Chair Cat Cow (Marjaryasana-Bitilasana)

This movement works the hips, the spine, the abdomen, and the shoulders.

1. Begin by sitting slightly forward and upright in your chair with your feet planted firmly on the ground.

2. Place your arms on your thighs.

3. Keep your gaze forward and your spine elongated.

4. Inhale and arch your back and push your chest forward. This is the cow position. Hold this for three to five breaths.

5. Return to your starting position.

6. Inhale and arch your back in the opposite direction with your chest moving inwards and

your back outwards. Hold this for three to five breaths.

7. Return to your starting position.

Chair Triangle Pose

This pose works your core as well as your hamstrings and hips.

1. Begin by sitting slightly forward and upright in your chair with your feet planted firmly on the ground. Your legs should be touching.

2. Place your hands on your thighs.

3. Keep your gaze forward and your spine elongated.

4. Inhale and raise your arms to your side so they are in line with your shoulders.

5. Gently exhale and twist, bringing your left hand down to your right ankle or as far as you feel comfortable.

6. Gently raise your right hand toward the ceiling at the same time. Look up toward this hand.

7. Hold for three breaths.

8. Return to your starting position with arms in line with shoulders.

9. Repeat on the other side.

Torso Rotation

This pose is very beneficial for your spine and lower back, but if you have spinal stenosis, disk herniations, or osteoporosis of the spine, you should skip this pose.

1. Begin by sitting slightly forward and upright in your chair with your feet planted firmly on the ground. Your legs should be touching.

2. Place your palms together in a prayer pose in front of your chest.

3. Keep your gaze forward and your spine elongated.

4. Inhale deeply, and as you exhale, twist your torso to the left.

5. Return to the center and repeat on the other side.

6. Repeat for 10 repetitions.

Seated Downward Facing Dog Pose

This widely recognized position opens up the chest and focuses on the lower and upper back muscles.

1. Begin by sitting slightly forward and upright in your chair with your feet planted firmly on the ground. Your legs should be about hip distance apart.

2. Place your hands on your thighs.

3. Keep your gaze forward and your spine elongated.

4. Stretch your legs out in front of you with your heels on the ground and your toes toward the ceiling.

5. Lengthen your spine as you inhale and press your heels into the floor.

6. Exhale as you lean your chest forward and raise your hands up and out in front of you in line with your ears. Spread your fingers wide, palms facing forward.

7. Press forward with your hands as if there is a wall in front of you and continue to press your heels to the floor.

8. Hold this position for three deep breaths.

9. Return to the starting position.

Chair Mountain Pose Standing Flow

This flow will target your whole body.

1. Begin by sitting upright in your chair with your feet planted firmly on the ground. The distance between your legs should be a fist wide and your knees should be directly over your ankles.

2. Place your arms on either side of you.

3. Keep your gaze forward and your spine elongated.

4. Inhale and stand up.

5. Exhale and sit back down.

6. Repeat for 10 repetitions.

Seated Hip Hinges

This targets your abdominal muscles as well as the surrounding muscles that make up your core.

1. Begin by sitting forward and upright in your chair with your feet planted firmly on the ground. Your legs should be about hip distance apart.

2. Cross your hands in front of your chest.

3. Keep your gaze forward and your spine elongated.

4. Keeping your back straight, gently inhale and lean back and tap the back of your chair with your shoulders.

5. Exhale and lift yourself forward again.

6. Focus on using your abdominal muscles to move you back and forth.

7. Repeat for 10 repetitions.

Modified Squat

This movement works the lower body as well as your midline. This is a great movement to use as a warm-up movement as well.

1. Begin by standing behind your chair and take a step back.

2. Place your feet directly underneath your hips and about shoulder-width apart with your toes turned slightly outwards.

3. Place your hands on the back of your chair for support and stability.

4. Inhale and gently push your hips back as if you are going to sit down.

5. Keep your knees behind your toes and push outwards.

6. Keep your shoulders back and your chest raised as you lower yourself to a comfortable depth.

7. Exhale and stand.

8. Repeat for 10 repetitions.

Seated Single Leg Extensions

This movement will work your midline as well as your hamstrings, quads, hips, and glutes.

1. Begin by sitting upright in your chair with your feet planted firmly on the ground. Your back should be up against the backrest of the chair.

2. Your legs should be about hip distance apart.

3. Place your hands on either side of the seat for stability.

4. Keep your gaze forward and your spine elongated.

5. Inhale and gently raise your left leg out in front of you, keeping your knee straight.

6. Raise it to a height where the leg remains straight but you are still comfortable.

7. Keep your right leg firmly planted on the ground.

8. Hold for two breaths.

9. Return to the neutral position.

10. Inhale and gently raise your right leg out in front of you, keeping your knee straight.

11. Raise it to a height where the leg remains straight but you are still comfortable.

12. Keep your left leg firmly planted on the ground.

13. Hold for two breaths.

14. Return to the neutral position.

15. Repeat for 10 alternating repetitions.

Chair Yoga Balance Exercises

These exercises will help improve your balance. Some of them are not yoga poses, but I have chosen to incorporate them as I feel they are of great benefit to us, and we can and should be using them in our practice.

Gait Awareness

This exercise improves body awareness and balance while we are moving.

1. Begin by sitting upright in your chair with your feet planted firmly on the ground.

2. Place your hands on your thighs.

3. Keep your gaze forward and your spine elongated.

4. Draw awareness to your feet and raise yourself to stand.

5. Slowly walk forward, paying attention to your foot positioning and pressure on the ground.

6. Walk back toward the chair and sit down.

7. Repeat five times.

Sit and Stands

This exercise helps with your balance as well as builds and maintains strength to help you sit and stand independently.

1. Begin by sitting slightly forward and upright in your chair with your feet planted firmly on the ground. Your legs should be about hip distance apart.

2. Place your hands on your thighs.

3. Keep your gaze forward and your spine elongated.

4. Engage your midline and tip slightly forward from your hips.

5. Draw awareness to your feet and push yourself to stand. Extend your knees and hips fully.

6. Gently reverse the movement by pushing your hips backward and lowering yourself to the chair.

Standing Triangle

This pose will work on your balance while you are in a unilateral position.

1. Stand sideways beside your chair with your feet three to four inches apart.

2. Point the toes of your foot that are closest to the chair toward the seat, and the foot furthest away should be at a 45° angle.

3. As you inhale, raise your arms to shoulder height, creating a T shape with your upper body.

4. As you exhale, lower the arm closest to the chair down and let it rest on either the seat or the back of the chair—whatever is most comfortable for you.

5. Hold for three breaths.

6. Repeat on the other side.

7. Return to the starting position.

Palm Tree

This pose will test your balance while you stand on your toes.

1. Stand upright while facing the back of your chair.

2. Take hold of the back of the chair and rise on the balls of your feet.

3. Lift your left arm overhead and hold for three breaths.

4. Return to the starting position.

5. Lift your right arm overhead and hold for three breaths.

Moving Crescent Moon

This pose will work on your balance as you transition between different movements.

1. Stand upright while facing the back of your chair.

2. Take hold of the back of the chair.

3. Raise your left hand upward, leaning slightly over your head while simultaneously shifting your weight to your right leg and raising that heel off the floor.

4. Return to the starting position.

5. Raise your right hand upward, leaning slightly over your head while simultaneously shifting your weight to your left leg and raising that heel off the floor.

6. Continue to gently flow from side to side for five to eight repetitions.

Chapter 6:

Moderate-Intensity Chair Yoga

Program

This exercise is a moderate-intensity program that is targeted toward those 60 years of age, but it can be used by anyone looking for a less strenuous workout or has certain limitations where this program will be better suited.

If you are capable, you can incorporate and perform poses from the previous chapter as well as this one—all sections can be customizable to meet you where you are at.

As usual, we will do a quick warm-up routine, then you may choose three to five poses for each specific muscle group that we will be focusing on during this session: the upper body, midsection, and lower body.

Warm-up

1. We will begin by lightly jogging on the spot for 30–60 seconds. If this is too strenuous, please

march on the spot instead or in a chair as per previous chapters.

2. Remain standing upright with your shoulders back and down, gently squeezing them toward each other. Hold for two breaths, then release.

3. Repeat these shoulder squeezes eight times.

4. Keep your feet hip-width apart and raise your hands over your head.

5. Slowly fold forward from your hips, moving vertebrae by vertebrae, and go down as low as you feel comfortable.

6. Hold for two breaths.

7. Slowly raise yourself back up from your hips, moving vertebrae by vertebrae, until you are upright with your hands over your head.

8. Repeat 10 times.

Chair Yoga Upper-Body Exercises

Down Dog on Chair (Uttana Shishosana)

This pose works the upper body and opens up your chest.

1. Stand behind your chair.

2. Place your hands on the back of your chair; they should be about shoulder-width apart.

3. Step backward until your legs are underneath your hips. You should create a right angle with your body and your back remains flat like a tabletop.

4. Ground and anchor your feet to the ground, lifting through your thighs.

5. Push your hips away from your hands. You should feel an elongation in the sides of your body.

6. Hold for five breaths.

Chair Chest Expansions

This pose concentrates on your chest muscles as well as your arms and shoulders.

1. Begin by sitting slightly forward and upright in your chair with your feet planted firmly on the ground.

2. Place your hands on your thighs.

3. Keep your gaze forward and your spine elongated.

4. Inhale and bring your hands above you.

5. Exhale and bring your arms behind your back and hold onto the sides of your chair.

6. Inhale and gently push your chest forward. Your back will be bending slightly.

7. Exhale and release.

8. Repeat five times.

Seated Cactus Arm Flow on Chair

This flow builds strength and increases flexibility in the upper back, chest, neck, arms, and shoulders.

1. Begin by sitting upright in your chair with your feet planted firmly on the ground.

2. Place your hands on your thighs.

3. Keep your gaze forward and your spine elongated.

4. Inhale as you bring your arms to shoulder height, keeping them bent at the elbows and your palms facing forward.

5. Exhale and spread your fingers out wide.

6. Inhale, and on your exhale, bring your hands together so your palms and forearms are touching.

7. Inhale and move your arms outwards again

8. Exhale and bring them back together again.

9. Repeat six times.

Eagle Pose on Chair (Garudasana)

The eagle pose benefits the upper back, arms, shoulders, and the knees.

1. Begin by sitting upright and forward in your chair with your feet planted firmly on the ground.

2. Place your hands on your thighs.

3. Keep your gaze forward and your spine elongated.

4. Cross your left leg over your right leg. If you can, tuck your left toes behind your right calf.

5. As you inhale, extend your arms out to the side of your body.

6. As you exhale, extend them out in front of you. Place your right arm under your left arm. Grab each shoulder with the opposite hand similar to hugging yourself.

7. Depending on your flexibility, you could continue to wrap your forearms around each other until your right fingers are joined with your left palm.

8. On your inhale, lift your elbows higher and look up and back down.

9. Exhale and squeeze your thighs together.

10. Hold for five breaths.

11. Return to the starting position and repeat on the other side.

Seated Backbend With Eagle Arms in Chair

This pose will work your shoulders, arms, biceps, triceps, and upper back.

1. Begin by sitting upright and forward in your chair with your feet planted firmly on the ground.

2. Place your hands on your thighs.

3. Keep your gaze forward and your spine elongated.

4. As you inhale, extend your arms out to the side of your body.

5. As you exhale, extend them out in front of you. Place your right arm under your left arm. Grab each shoulder with the opposite hand similar to hugging yourself.

6. Depending on your flexibility, you could continue to wrap your forearms around each other until your right fingers are joined with your left palm.

7. On your inhale, lift your elbows higher and look up and back down.

8. Exhale and lean back and arch your back slightly.

9. Hold for three breaths.

10. Return to the starting position and swap arms.

Standing Lateral Side Bend

This pose is great for your upper body, particularly your

upper and middle back and chest.

1. Begin by standing behind or next to your chair. Your feet should be a hip distance apart.

2. Place your left palm on the back of your chair for support.

3. Inhale as you raise your right arm overhead.

4. As you gently exhale, lean toward the left, keeping both feet on the ground, your body in a straight line, and your hips aligned.

5. Keep your head facing forward and then bend it to the left and gaze toward your right hand.

6. Inhale as you focus on lengthening your spine, and exhale as you deepen the stretch.

7. Stay in this position for five breaths.

8. Return to the starting position.

9. Place your right palm on the back of your chair for support.

10. Inhale as you raise your left arm overhead.

11. As you gently exhale, lean toward the right, keeping both feet on the ground, your body in a straight line, and your hips aligned.

12. Keep your head facing forward and then bend it to the left and gaze toward your left hand.

13. Inhale as you focus on lengthening your spine, and exhale as you deepen the stretch.

14. Stay in this position for five breaths.

15. Return to the starting position.

Seated Arm Rotations

This movement works the shoulders and arms.

1. Begin by sitting upright in your chair with your feet planted firmly on the ground.

2. Place your hands on your thighs.

3. Keep your gaze forward and your spine elongated.

4. Bring your arms up and out to the side as you inhale deeply.

5. Exhale as they relax in line with your shoulders.

6. Begin to rotate them forward from your shoulders. Begin with small circles and slowly increase their size as you rotate them for 20 repetitions.

7. Return to the center.

8. Bring your arms up and out to the side as you inhale deeply.

9. Exhale as they relax in line with your shoulders.

10. Begin to rotate them backward from your shoulders. Begin with small circles and slowly increase their size as you rotate them for 20 repetitions.

11. Return to the center.

Chair Cobra Pose

This pose works the chest and upper back.

1. Begin by sitting upright on the front of your chair with your feet planted firmly on the ground.

2. Keep your gaze forward and your spine elongated.

3. Inhale and place your hands behind you and hold on to the edges of the seat of the chair.

4. Inhale and raise your chest and shoulders so you are looking upwards and there is a slight arch in your back.

5. Exhale and embrace the stretch.

6. Stay in this position for six breaths.

7. Relax and return to the neutral position.

Chair Yoga Lower-Body Exercises

These exercises will target your lower body. The main muscles we will be focusing on are the calves, quadriceps, hamstrings, and glutes.

Half-Seated Forward Bend

This pose will target your feet, ankles, hamstrings, and quads.

1. Begin by sitting upright and forward in your chair with your feet planted firmly on the ground.

2. Place your hands on your thighs.

3. Keep your gaze forward and your spine elongated.

4. Inhale, and on your exhale, stretch your right leg forward, extending your foot and resting it on its heel. Your toes should be pointing upwards as your feet are flexed.

5. Inhale, and as you exhale, bend forward from your waist. You should feel a stretch in your hamstrings and calves.

6. Hold for five breaths.

7. Return to the starting position.

8. Inhale, and on your exhale, stretch your left leg forward, extending your foot and resting it on its heel. Your toes should be pointing upwards as your feet are flexed.

9. Inhale, and as you exhale, bend forward from your waist. You should feel a stretch in your hamstrings and calves.

10. Hold for five breaths.

11. Return to the starting position.

Chair Pigeon Pose With Prayer Hands

This is a great pose for those of you with tight hips and glutes. It also targets the hamstrings and ankles.

1. Begin by sitting slightly forward and upright in your chair with your feet planted firmly on the ground.

2. Place your arms on either side of you.

3. Keep your gaze forward and your spine elongated.

4. Rest your left ankle on the top of your right knee.

5. Bring your palms together in front of your chest in a prayer position.

6. Inhale, and on your exhale, fold forward from your hips, keeping your back straight.

7. Take five breaths in this position and return to the starting position.

8. Rest your right ankle on the top of your left knee.

9. Bring your palms together in front of your chest in a prayer position.

10. Inhale, and on your exhale, fold forward from your hips, keeping your back straight.

11. Take five breaths in this position and return to the starting position.

Knee Lifts

These movements will work your quads, glutes, and knees.

1. Begin by sitting upright and forward in your chair

with your feet planted firmly on the ground.

2. Place your hands on your thighs.

3. Keep your gaze forward and your spine elongated.

4. Inhale and bring your left knee up toward your chest.

5. Pause for a five-second count.

6. Exhale and lower your leg.

7. Inhale and bring your right knee up toward your chest.

8. Pause for a five-second count.

9. Exhale and lower your leg.

10. Alternate and repeat 20 times.

Heel Slides

Heel slides target your quads, hamstrings, and calves.

1. Begin by sitting upright and forward in your chair with your feet planted firmly on the ground.

2. Place your hands on the edge of your chair for stability.

3. Keep your gaze forward and your spine elongated.

4. Point the toes of your left food out in front of you, and as you exhale, gently slide it forward.

5. Inhale and slide your left foot back toward you, keeping your sole flat on the ground.

6. Return to the starting position.

7. Point the toes on your right foot out in front of you, and as you exhale, gently slide it forward.

8. Inhale and slide your left foot back toward you, keeping your sole flat on the ground.

9. Return to the starting position.

10. Alternate feet and repeat 20 times.

Seated Low Lunge Variation (Anjaneyasana)

This pose targets your glutes and your knees.

1. Begin by sitting upright and forward in your chair with your feet planted firmly on the ground.

2. Place your hands on your thighs.

3. Keep your gaze forward and your spine elongated.

4. Inhale and bring your right knee up toward your chest as far as you are comfortable.

5. Wrap your arms around your leg to keep it in position.

6. Hold for three breaths.

7. Exhale and release.

8. Inhale and bring your left knee up toward your chest as far as you are comfortable.

9. Wrap your arms around your leg to keep it in position.

10. Hold for three breaths.

11. Exhale and release.

Chair Heel Raises

This movement targets all the muscles in the lower body, specifically the calves.

1. Stand behind your chair.

2. Place your hands on the back of your chair; they should be about shoulder-width apart.

3. Inhale and rise onto your toes.

4. Hold for six breaths and release.

5. Repeat 20 times.

Chair Mountain Pose With Raised Leg

This pose works the whole lower body. It targets the back, glutes, hamstrings, hips, feet, and ankles.

1. Stand behind your chair. Your feet should be hip distance apart and your arms should be almost straight.

2. Place your hands on the back of your chair. They should be about shoulder-width apart.

3. Inhale and raise your right leg behind you, bending slightly forward from your waist.

4. Hold for three breaths.

5. Return to the starting position.

6. Inhale and raise your left leg behind you, bending slightly forward from your waist.

7. Hold for three breaths.

8. Return to the starting position.

Chair Standing Twist

This pose targets your lower back, hips, glutes, and hamstrings.

1. Stand facing your chair. Your feet should be a hip distance apart.

2. Raise your right foot so it is resting on the chair. You will have created a 90° angle with your leg.

3. Your left leg should be underneath your left hip with your toes pointed toward the chair.

4. Place your left hand on the outside of your right knee.

5. Place your right hand on your lower back.

6. Inhale as you lengthen your spine.

7. Exhale and draw your belly button to your spine.

8. Inhale and gently twist from your midline.

9. Hold this position for five breaths.

10. Exhale and return to the starting position.

11. Raise your left foot so it is fully resting on the chair.

12. Your right leg should be underneath your left hip with your toes pointed toward the chair.

13. Place your right hand on the outside of your left knee.

14. Place your left hand on your lower back.

15. Inhale as you lengthen your spine.

16. Exhale and draw your belly button to your spine.

17. Inhale and gently twist from your midline.

18. Hold this position for five breaths.

Seated Windshield Wiper

This movement focuses on your hips, knees, and pelvis.

1. Begin by sitting upright and forward in your chair with your feet planted firmly on the ground. Your feet should be positioned a little more than hip-width apart.

2. Place your hands on the sides of the chair.

3. Keep your gaze forward and your spine elongated.

4. Inhale and drop your knees to the right.

5. Inhale and return to the center.

6. Exhale and drop your knees to the left.

7. Repeat for 20 repetitions.

Standing Gate Pose

The list of muscles that this pose works is extensive. This pose works your arms, shoulders, back, chest, core, glutes, hamstrings, hips, pelvis, knees, feet, ankles, and quads.

1. Begin by standing next to your chair.

2. Stretch your right leg out so your heel rests on the seat of your chair. Your knees and toes should be pointing upwards.

3. Raise your arms to your side, parallel to the floor with your palms facing upwards.

4. Inhale and lengthen.

5. Exhale and lower your right arm and body to your right leg. Keep your hips facing forward.

6. Rest your right arm on your right shin or ankle.

7. At the same time, bring your left arm up and reach over your head.

8. Hold for five to ten breaths.

9. Return to the center.

10. Turn around so the chair is now on your left side.

11. Stretch your left leg out so your heel rests on the seat of your chair. Your knees and toes should be pointing upwards.

12. Raise your arms to your side, parallel to the floor with your palms facing upwards.

13. Inhale and lengthen.

14. Exhale and lower your left arm and body to your left leg. Keep your hips facing forward.

15. Rest your left arm on your left shin or ankle.

16. At the same time, bring your right arm up and reach over your head.

17. Hold for five to ten breaths.

18. Return to the center.

Chair Yoga Full-Body Exercises

These exercises will target your torso and midline, which includes your core and lower and upper back. The main muscles we will be focusing on are the abdominal core muscles and back.

Revolved Chair Pose (Parivrtta Utkatasana)

This pose is a full-body pose and works your neck, arms, shoulders, chest, upper and lower back, as well as your psoas.

1. Begin by sitting upright in your chair with your feet planted firmly on the ground.

2. Place your hands on your thighs.

3. Keep your gaze forward and your spine elongated.

4. Bend forward from your hips and place your right elbow and forearm along your right and left knees.

5. Take a deep inhale, and as you exhale, turn your body to the left.

6. Reach your left hand to the ceiling and allow your gaze to follow your left hand.

7. Hold for three deep breaths.

8. Return to your starting position and repeat on the other side.

Captain's Chair

This exercise will strengthen your abdominal and back muscles as well as your glutes.

1. Begin by sitting upright in your chair with your feet planted firmly on the ground.

2. Place your hands on either side of the edge of your seat.

3. Keep your gaze forward and your spine elongated.

4. Inhale and slowly lift your feet off the floor, moving your knees toward your chest. Raise them as far as you feel comfortable.

5. Exhale and slowly lower them.

6. Repeat 10 times.

Three-Legged Downward Dog

This variation of the downward dog targets the lower back, core, hamstring, and hips.

1. Begin by standing behind your chair. Your feet should be hip distance apart and your arms should be almost straight.

2. Place your hands on the back of your chair. They should be about shoulder-width apart.

3. Step backward until your legs are underneath your hips. You should create a right angle with your body and your back remains flat like a tabletop.

4. Ground and anchor your feet to the ground, lifting through your thighs.

5. Push your hips away from your hands. You should feel an elongation in the sides of your body.

6. Lift your left leg out behind you, keeping it as straight as you can.

7. Hold for three breaths.

8. Return to the starting position.

9. Lift your right leg out behind you, keeping it as straight as you can.

10. Return to the starting position.

11. Repeat 10 times.

Goddess Pose on Chair

This pose works your arms, triceps, biceps, hips, knees, and pelvis.

1. Begin by sitting upright in your chair with your feet planted firmly on the ground.

2. Place your hands on your thighs.

3. Keep your gaze forward and your spine elongated.

4. Widen your legs, turning your feet outwards. Keep your toes in line with your feet.

5. Inhale and bring your arms up over your head.

6. Exhale and bring them down so they are in line with your shoulders and your elbows are bent at a 90° angle.

7. Your palms should be facing forward with your fingers spread wide.

8. Hold this for five to ten breaths.

Wide-Legged Seated Twist

This pose targets your hips, knees, chest, back, as well as your shoulders and arms.

1. Begin by sitting upright in your chair with your feet planted firmly on the ground.

2. Place your hands on your thighs.

3. Keep your gaze forward and your spine elongated.

4. Widen your legs, turning your feet outwards. Keep your toes in line with your feet.

5. Inhale and twist from your torso to the right.

6. Bring your left arm to rest on your right thigh.

7. Hold for three breaths.

8. Return to the starting position.

9. Inhale and twist from your torso to the left.

10. Bring your right arm to rest on your left thigh.

11. Hold for three breaths.

12. Return to the starting position.

Chair Yoga Balance Exercises

These accessory exercises will help improve your balance. I suggest adding them to your warm-up or cooldown routines.

Single Leg Balance

1. Begin by standing behind your chair. Your feet should be hip distance apart and your arms should be almost straight.

2. Place your hands on the back of your chair for support.

3. Slowly lift your left leg off the floor by bending the knee up toward your chest.

4. Straighten your left leg in front of you and hold in this position for 30 seconds.

5. Return to the starting position.

6. Slowly lift your right leg off the floor by bending the knee up toward your chest.

7. Straighten your right leg in front of you and hold in this position for 30 seconds.

8. Return to the starting position.

Tightrope Walk

1. Stand up in front of the straight line you are going to use as your reference point for a tightrope. You could mark out a line on the floor using painter's tape or you could use the edge of a rug or your floor tiles.

2. Extend your arms out to the side for balance.

3. Begin to walk slowly, from heel to toe, along the line.

4. Count for five seconds between each step.

Tree Pose

1. Begin by standing behind or next to your chair. Your feet should be a hip distance apart.

2. Place your hand on the back of your chair for support.

3. Shifting your weight onto your right foot, gently raise your left foot and place the sole against the inner calf of your left leg.

4. The knee of your right leg will be turned outwards, your hips and body facing forward.

5. If you are capable, bring both palms together in a praying position and hold for three breaths.

6. Return to the starting position.

7. Repeat on the other side.

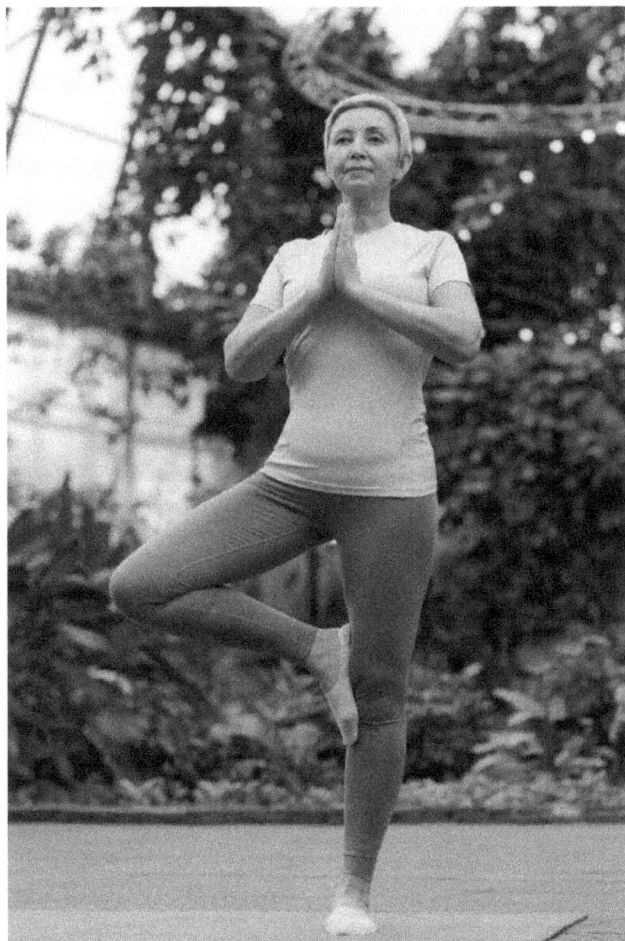

Chapter 7:

High-Intensity Chair Yoga

Program

The next chapter will introduce you to slightly more advanced poses and movements that you can use to make your practice more challenging.

Again, you can pick and choose any movement, pose, or balance exercise from any chapter to create a varied routine. You can also modify any exercise to make them more or less difficult for you.

Warm-up

1. We will begin with jumping jacks. These can be done standing in front of or sitting on a chair depending on your fitness level. Perform for 30 seconds.

2. Standing upright with your shoulders back and down, gently tilt your right ear toward your right shoulder and feel the stretch. Hold for three breaths.

3. Return to the starting position and repeat on the left side.

4. Repeat 10 times.

5. Remain standing and place your fingertips on your shoulders. Rotate your shoulders forward for 10 repetitions.

6. Return to the starting position and rotate your shoulders backward for 10 repetitions.

7. Keep your feet hip-width apart and raise your hands over your head.

8. Slowly fold forward from your hips, moving vertebrae by vertebrae as low as you feel comfortable.

9. Hold for two breaths.

10. Slowly raise yourself back up from your hips, moving vertebrae by vertebrae until you are upright with your hands over your head.

11. Repeat 10 times.

12. Place your hands on your waist.

13. Moving from your waist, circle your hips five times clockwise then circle your hips five times counterclockwise.

14. Repeat three times.

Chair Yoga Upper-Body Exercises

These are more intensive movements that will challenge your upper body. This includes your arms, shoulders, biceps, triceps, forearms, upper back, and chest.

Puppy Dog Pose on Chair

This pose centers around your arms and shoulders, upper back, and chest.

1. Begin by standing in front of your chair. Your feet should be hip-width apart.

2. Gently come down into a kneeling position, facing the front of your chair. You should be able to stretch your arms out straight in front of you and rest your palms on the front of the chair.

3. Your knees should be in line with your hips, creating a 90° angle, and your back should be flat.

4. Slowly press your chest downwards toward the ground, feeling a stretch along the side of your body.

5. Hold for five breaths.

Seated Five-Pointed Star Pose

This pose will work your arms, shoulders, upper back, and chest muscles.

1. Begin by sitting upright in your chair with your feet planted firmly on the ground.

2. Place your hands on your thighs.

3. Keep your gaze forward and your spine elongated.

4. Slightly tuck in your chin.

5. Roll your shoulder blades back and down, activating your upper back muscles.

6. Inhale and lift your arms to the side and overhead creating a Y shape.

7. Exhale and lower them back down to your side.

8. Repeat for 15 repetitions.

Dolphin Pose on Chair

The dolphin pose is used to build strength and flexibility in your arms, shoulders, and middle and upper back.

1. Begin by standing in front of your chair. Your feet should be hip-width apart.

2. Facing the front of your chair, bend gently at your hips so your forearms are resting on the seat of your chair.

3. Your arms should be shoulder-width apart with your head in between your elbows.

4. If you can manage it, rest your forehead on the seat.

5. Hold for five breaths.

6. Return to standing.

Chair Sun Breaths

This sequence is a dynamic movement that works your arms.

1. Begin by sitting upright in your chair with your feet planted firmly on the ground.

2. Place your hands on your thighs.

3. Keep your gaze forward and your spine elongated.

4. Inhale and reach your arms overhead.

5. Exhale and bar your palms together at the center of your chest. Pause for one breath.

6. Repeat five to ten times.

Head up Chair Pose

This pose focuses on the neck.

1. Begin by sitting upright in your chair with your feet planted firmly on the ground.

2. Place your hands on either side of the seat of your chair.

3. Keep your gaze forward and your spine elongated.

4. Inhale and extend your arms upwards and forward.

5. Exhale and bend from the hips and bring your arms toward your shins.

6. Let your hands rest comfortably on your shins.

7. Tilt your chin upwards.

8. Hold for four breaths.

9. Inhale and return to the starting position.

Chair Yoga Lower-Body Exercises

These exercises will target your lower body. The main muscles we will be focusing on are the calves, quadriceps, hamstrings, and glutes.

Chair High Lunge

This pose targets your glutes, hamstrings, hips, and knees.

1. Stand behind your chair. Your feet should be a hip distance apart.

2. Place your hands on the back of your chair. They should be about shoulder-width apart.

3. Take a step backward with your left leg.

4. Slowly lower your left knee toward the ground.

5. Your front knee will also bend, and it should be directly in line with your ankle and foot.

6. Keep both feet flat on the ground and hold for five breaths.

7. Return to the starting position.

8. Repeat on the other side.

Standing Tabletop Pose With Knee to Nose Flow

This pose works your lower back, core, glutes, hamstrings, hips, knees, and quads.

1. Begin by standing in front of your chair. Your feet should be hip-distance apart.

2. Rest your palms on the front seat of your chair, bending from your hips.

3. Inhale and extend your left leg out behind you. Extend it as far out as you feel comfortable.

4. Exhale and bring your knee toward your chest.

5. Repeat for 10 repetitions.

6. Return to the starting position and repeat on the other side.

Easy Pose to Chair Pose

This pose targets your glutes and quads.

1. Begin by sitting upright in your chair with your feet planted firmly on the ground.

2. Place your hands on either side of the seat of your chair.

3. Keep your gaze forward and your spine elongated.

4. Inhale and shift your weight forward, and slowly raise your hips off the chair. Do not stand up fully but remain half seated, half standing.

5. Keep your knees bent and your head facing forward.

6. Exhale and return to your seated position.

7. Repeat 10 times.

Seated Hip Circles

This movement focuses on your pelvis and hips.

1. Begin by sitting upright in your chair with your feet planted firmly on the ground.

2. Place your hands on either side of the seat of your chair.

3. Keep your gaze forward and your spine elongated.

4. Inhale and slowly begin to rotate your torso in a clockwise direction.

5. Begin with small circles and increase them as you continue to move.

6. Repeat for 20 circles in a clockwise direction.

7. Return to the starting position.

8. Repeat in an anticlockwise direction for 20 repetitions.

Mountain Pose to Chair Pose

This pose works your lower back and quads.

1. Stand behind your chair. Your feet should be hip-distance apart, and your arms should be almost straight.

2. Place your hands on the back of your chair. They should be about shoulder-width apart.

3. Inhale and stand up tall, extend your spine upwards, and relax your shoulders.

4. Exhale and push your hips back into a half-sitting position, bringing your weight into your heels.

5. Your knees should be behind your toes.

6. Keep your back straight.

7. Hold for three breaths.

8. Return to a standing position.

9. Repeat five times.

Intense Side Stretch Pose With Hands on Chair

This is a great pose for your lower body as it works your middle back, lower back, hamstrings, hips, and pelvis.

1. Begin by standing in front of your chair. Your feet should be a hip distance apart.

2. You want to stand just far enough away to be able to reach the middle of the seat with flat hands when you bend over.

3. Bring your right foot forward and position it just under the chair. Keep your right knee straight.

4. Keep your left heel on the ground with your toes turned slightly upwards.

5. Exhale and bend from your hips and place both palms on the seat of the chair.

6. Push your hips back, creating a stretch in your hamstrings.

7. Hold for five breaths.

8. Return to standing.

9. Bring your left foot forward and position it just under the chair. Keep your left knee straight.

10. Keep your right heel on the ground with your toes turned slightly upwards.

11. Exhale and bend from your hips and place both palms on the seat of the chair.

12. Push your hips back, creating a stretch in your hamstrings.

13. Hold for five breaths.

14. Return to standing.

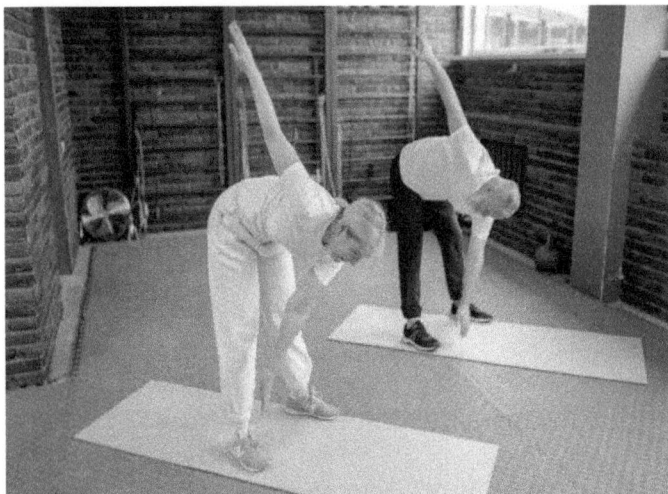

Seated Straddle Pose

This pose focuses on the lower back, glutes, hips, pelvis, and quads.

1. Begin by sitting down facing the front of your chair. Your legs should be wide apart at a comfortable distance.

2. Your knees and toes should be facing the ceiling.

3. Inhale and lengthen up through your spine.

4. As you exhale, bend forward from your hips, resting your forearms on the chair and your head on your forearms.

5. Hold for two to five minutes and progressively deepen the stretch.

Bound Angle Chair Pose

This pose focuses on your lower back and pelvis.

1. Begin by sitting down facing the front of your chair.

2. Bring the soles of your feet together. If you cannot manage this, then sit cross-legged.

3. Place your arms on the seat of your chair and gently fold forward and place your head on your arms.

4. Hold for two to five minutes and progressively deepen the stretch.

Chair Staff Pose

This pose works your hamstrings, hips, and quads.

1. Begin by sitting upright in your chair with your feet planted firmly on the ground.

2. Place your hands on either side of the seat of your chair.

3. Keep your gaze forward and your spine elongated.

4. Engage your abdominals.

5. Inhale and raise both your legs out in front of you.

6. Keep your legs straight and flex your feet upwards, your toes pointing back toward you and your heels away from you.

7. Hold for three breaths.

8. On your last exhale, lower your legs and return to the starting position.

Chair Yoga Full-Body Exercises

These exercises will target your torso and midline, which includes your core and lower and upper back. The main muscles we will be focusing on are the abdominal core muscles and back.

Seated Revolved Arms With Extended Eagle Legs

This pose targets most of the muscles in your body, including your arms and shoulders, upper and middle back, hamstrings, chest, hips, knees, pelvis, psoas, and quads.

1. Begin by sitting upright and slightly forward in your chair with your feet planted firmly on the ground.

2. Place your hands on either side of the seat of your chair.

3. Keep your gaze forward and your spine elongated.

4. Cross your right leg over your left leg with your lower leg hanging freely on the other side.

5. Raise your arms and extend them out to your side, keeping them straight and in line with your shoulders.

6. Exhale as you gently twist and turn your gaze to your left.

7. Hold for five breaths.

8. Return to the center.

9. Cross your left leg over your right leg with your lower leg hanging freely on the other side.

10. Raise your arms and extend them out to your side, keeping them straight and in line with your shoulders.

11. Exhale as you gently twist and turn your gaze to your right.

12. Hold for five breaths.

13. Return to the center.

Extended Side Angle Pose Variation

This pose targets most of the muscles in your body, including the core, hamstrings, chest, hips, knees, pelvis, psoas, and quads.

1. Begin by sitting upright and slightly forward in your chair with your feet planted firmly on the ground.

2. Place your hands on either side of the seat of your chair.

3. Keep your gaze forward and your spine elongated.

4. Position yourself so that you are seated slightly sideways so your left thigh is resting across the seat of your chair.

5. Stretch out your right leg, straightening your knees and ankles.

6. While you inhale, gently raise your right arm above your head.

7. While placing your left forearm on your left thigh, exhale.

8. Hold this position for three breaths.

9. Release and return to the starting position.

10. Reposition yourself so you are seated slightly sideways so your right thigh is resting across the seat of your chair.

11. Stretch out your left leg, straightening your knees and ankles.

12. While you inhale, gently raise your left arm above your head.

13. While placing your right forearm on your left thigh, exhale.

14. Hold this position for three breaths.

15. Release and return to the starting position.

Chair Plank

This exercise targets your core and midline, which is your abdominal muscles and lower back muscles.

1. Begin by standing in front of your chair. Your feet should be a hip distance apart.

2. Place both hands on the side of the seat.

3. Keep your arms slightly bent at the elbows and walk yourself backward until your body is in a diagonal position.

4. Do not arch your back, and make sure your buttocks is not too high in the air. Your back should be flat and your body in a straight line.

5. Hold this position for 30 seconds (or however long you can manage).

6. Rest.

7. Repeat two to three times.

Boat Pose on Chair

This pose works your core muscles and builds midline strength. It is a great exercise for your abdominal muscles and quads.

1. Begin by sitting upright and forward in your chair with your feet planted firmly on the ground.

2. Place your hands on either side of the seat of your chair.

3. Keep your gaze forward and your spine elongated.

4. Inhale and bring your legs up so you are leaning backward slightly as you do so. You can do this one leg at a time if need be.

5. Exhale and bend your knees toward your chest.

6. Adjust your positioning so you are stable and comfortable on the chair.

7. Hold this position for two to three breaths.

8. Return to the starting position.

Dancer Pose

This pose works your whole body. It focuses on the arms, upper back, biceps, triceps, feet, ankles, hamstrings, chest, and hips.

1. Begin by standing behind your chair. Your feet should be a hip distance apart.

2. Place your hands on the back of your chair. They should be about shoulder-width apart.

3. Inhale and bend your left leg behind you and grab your left ankle with your left hand.

4. Exhale as you stretch your leg out as far as you feel comfortable.

5. Keep your hips square as you hold this for three breaths.

6. Release and return to the starting position.

7. Repeat on the other side.

Revolved Goddess Pose

This is a full-body pose. The muscles targeted here are the arms, shoulders, chest, midline, back, hamstrings, knees, pelvis, quads, wrists, and psoas.

1. Begin by sitting upright and forward in your chair with your feet planted firmly on the ground.

2. Place your hands on either side of the seat of your chair.

3. Keep your gaze forward and your spine elongated.

4. Open your legs wide, toes turned outwards with your knees in line with your feet.

5. Bending from your hips, exhale and bring your right arm down to the ground in between your feet.

6. Inhale and twist your body to bring your left arm up over your head.

7. Keep your gaze toward your left hand.

8. Stretch your fingers toward the sky.

9. Hold for three breaths.

10. Return to the starting position.

11. Repeat on the other side.

Goddess Pose Flow on Chair

Just like the Revolved Goddess Pose above, this flow will work the arms, shoulders, chest, midline, back, hamstrings, knees, pelvis, quads, wrists, and psoas.

1. Begin by sitting upright and forward in your chair with your feet planted firmly on the ground.

2. Keep your gaze forward and your spine elongated.

3. Inhale and open your legs wide, toes turned outwards with your knees in line with your feet. Your feet should be firmly planted on the ground. Shift forward in your chair if needed.

4. Place your hands on your thighs.

5. As you inhale, raise your arms overhead, shoulder-width apart, with palms facing each other. Hold for 30 seconds.

6. As you exhale, bring your arms down to shoulder level, keeping the elbows bent and creating a 90° angle with your arms. Hold for 30 seconds.

7. Squeeze your shoulder blades together.

8. Inhale and extend the arms up, lifting them overhead with palms facing each other. Hold for 30 seconds.

9. Exhale and lower your arms and place them on your inner thighs. Hold for 30 seconds.

10. Repeat for two to three minutes.

Standing Cat Cow Pose

This pose works your lower back and your core muscles in your midline.

1. Begin by standing in front of your chair. Your feet should be a hip distance apart.

2. Place both hands on the side of the seat.

3. Align your shoulders over your wrists and your hips over your feet.

4. Inhale and tilt your hips upwards.

5. Drop your belly and slightly raise your chest and head.

6. Hold for three breaths.

7. Exhale and tilt your hips downward.

8. Push your shoulder blades upwards and together, rounding the top of your back.

9. Hold for three breaths.

Corpse Pose With Chair

This is a restorative post that targets your whole body.

1. Begin by standing in front of your chair. Your feet should be hip-width apart.

2. Gently lower yourself onto your back and place your calves onto the seat of the chair. Your hips will be directly under your knees, creating a 90° angle.

3. Bring your arms to either side of you with the palms facing the ground.

4. Hold this position for 10 breaths.

Gate Pose on Chair

This is a full-body pose. The muscles targeted here are the arms, shoulders, chest, midline, back, hamstrings, knees, pelvis, and quads.

1. Begin by sitting upright and forward in your chair with your feet planted firmly on the ground.

2. Place your hands on either side of the seat of your chair.

3. Keep your gaze forward and your spine elongated.

4. As you inhale, extend your right leg outwards.

5. Exhale and place your left foot firmly on the floor.

6. Inhale and lift your left arm toward the ceiling. Raise it above and over your head, stretching slightly.

7. Exhale as you extend your right hand down and rest it on your knee or the side of your shin.

8. Hold for three breaths while actively deepening the stretch.

9. Return to the starting position.

10. Inhale and extend your left leg outwards.

11. Exhale and place your right foot firmly on the floor.

12. Inhale and lift your right arm toward the ceiling. Raise it above and over your head, stretching slightly.

13. Exhale as you extend your left hand down and rest it on your knee or the side of your shin.

14. Hold for three breaths while actively deepening the stretch.

15. Return to the starting position.

Chair Yoga Balance Exercises

Standing Split Chair Pose

1. Begin by standing in front of your chair. Your feet should be a hip distance apart.

2. Bring the right heel of your right foot onto the seat of the chair.

3. Keep your leg straight with your weight on your left foot and your hips square to the chair.

4. Hold for five breaths.

5. Return to the starting position.

6. Repeat on the other side.

Heel to Toe Walk

1. Begin by standing tall.

2. Slowly and deliberately place your right foot in front of your left foot.

3. Touch your right heel to your left toe.

4. Then place your left foot in front of your right foot.

5. Touch your left heel to your right toe.

6. Repeat for 20 steps.

Forward Toe Walking

1. Begin by standing tall next to your chair.

2. Raise onto the toes of your feet. You can use your chair for support.

3. Slowly walk forward using small steps. Keep your steps small and deliberate, and do not step through. Meet both feet in the middle, and then take a step.

4. Once you have walked 10 paces, begin to walk backward. Again, take a step so that both feet are together, then step back and away.

5. Repeat three times.

Moving Crescent Moon

1. Begin by standing behind your chair. Your feet should be a hip distance apart.

2. Place your hands on the back of your chair. They should be about shoulder-width apart.

3. Inhale and reach your left hand upwards and shift your weight to the right foot.

4. Lift your left heel off the floor.

5. Exhale and bring your arms back to the center and stand with both feet back on the floor.

6. Inhale and repeat on the other side.

7. Repeat this for 20 alternating repetitions.

Rock the Boat

1. Begin by standing tall next to your chair with your feet hip-distance apart.

2. You can use the chair for support, but if you feel comfortable, lift both your arms to the side and extend them outwards.

3. Lift your right foot off the floor and bend your knee, bringing your right heel toward your bottom.

4. Hold this position for 30 seconds.

5. Return to the starting position.

6. Lift your left foot off the floor and bend your knee, bringing your left heel toward your bottom.

7. Hold this position for 30 seconds.

8. Return to the starting position.

We have gone through three different levels of poses, movements, and exercises ranging from the low intensity, middle intensity, and high intensity. They are all classified based on their particular function and the muscles that they target. You have a lot of information to create a wonderful chair yoga workout program for yourself.

These movements and poses can be interchanged easily, so you do not need to stick to only low-intensity movements when creating a plan for yourself. Please mix it up if you feel you are capable.

I encourage you to stick to warming up first and then selecting about three to five exercises per muscle group as a template for your workouts. You will ensure you are prepared for your exercise, as well as give your whole body a good workout and not neglect any muscle groups.

Your balancing exercises can either be done as part of your warm-up or your cooldown. I would suggest mixing them up depending on how you feel.

If your chair yoga session was rather light and easy on you, then incorporate the balance exercises into your cool down. This ensures you will not be too tired to complete them properly but exhausted enough to make them more of a challenge. If you think your yoga program for the day may be too intense that the movements become too difficult, then use them as warm-up movements.

Whatever route you take with your program, remember to do it with intention.

Conclusion

You have heard of the phrase *life span*, but are you familiar with the *health span?* Life span is how long we will live, and our health span is how many of those years will be spent living in a healthy state.

We want to extend both of those. We want our health span to run parallel to our life span, ensuring we are free from diseases and other factors that contribute to ill health. There is no use in getting older if the quality of our life is poor and we cannot enjoy these years.

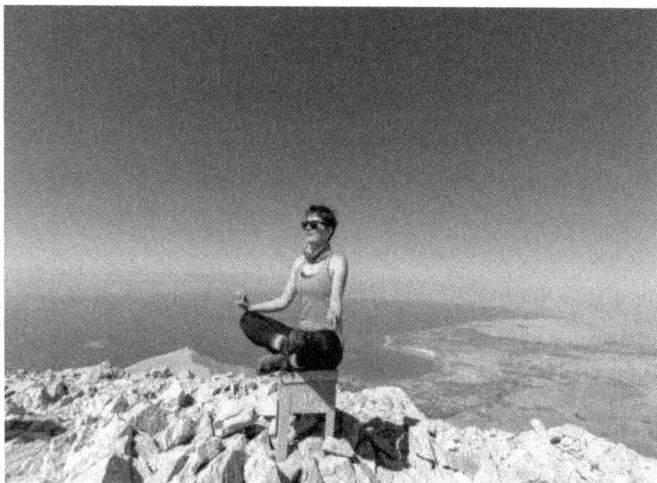

You have taken an important step in preserving or adding to your health span. Congratulations on taking control and altering your life path. Not many are brave enough to do it as they get older, and it is often to our detriment.

As we age and our lives change, we tend to accept our physical and mental limitations. This cycle continues as we make choices based on our perceived limitations, resulting in us taking on far less stimulating activities and projects as we feel these are within our reduced capabilities to complete.

We begin to do less and less. Emanuel (2014) uses an analogy of a canvas, which I think sums the idea up perfectly. We want to continue to paint, but we make the canvas smaller.

You have made your canvas bigger by choosing to work on your physical and mental health, using yoga as the vessel to accomplish and maintain wellness as you age.

I hope that this book becomes a well-worn companion for you. I have just scratched the surface of yoga and its poses, history, and intentions, but I believe that for most of you, this will be enough to spark your curiosity to dive deeper into its world.

Glossary

Adi Guru: The first guru or spiritual teacher.

Adiyogi: The first yogi.

Asana: The literal translation is seat, but it is interpreted as poses and postures.

Ashram: A yoga retreat.

Ashtanga: This type of yoga makes use of a continuous flow throughout the practice. This type of yoga is also considered more athletic. It consists of a series of 26 postures and was created by Bikram Choudhury.

Bhagavad Gita: The sacred Sanskrit text of yoga.

Bhanda: A muscular lock or seal. When these muscles are engaged, they tone, support, and promote energy flow. There are three main locks: Mula Bandha (root lock), Uddiyana Bandha (naval lock), and Jalandhara Bandha (throat lock).

Bikram Yoga: This yoga is practiced in a hot room that is usually 105°F

Block: A block is a yoga prop that helps yogis get into particular poses.

Chakra: The chakras are the energy centers of the body. The translation is a wheel, and there are seven chakras in the body, which have an association with particular colors, emotions, and elements. The seven chakras are the root, the sacral, the solar plexus, the heart, the throat, the third eye, and the crown.

Chaturanga: This is a pose that is performed on four limbs. It is similar to a staff pose or low plank.

Core: The core comprises muscles that wrap around your midlines, such as your abdominals and back muscles.

Dharma: Your path and purpose in life.

Drishti: Drishti is the area where you focus when you gaze during meditation or practice.

Guru: A mentor, guide, teacher, or master. This is a Sanskrit term.

Hatha: Refers to yoga for the physical body. It is the most basic style of yoga and is the basis for most of the different styles of yoga. It is usually slower-paced.

Heart Center: The term used to refer to the chest area.

Integrative Yoga: This practice was developed for medical settings. It is the use of yoga as a complementary treatment alongside others. It has been used on patients with cardiac problems and AIDS.

Iyengar Yoga: This yoga is ideal for those injured or who require less intensive practice. It uses props such as chairs, blocks, bands, belts, and blankets. These poses are held for much longer, and the mind-muscle connection is strongly emphasized.

Karma: This is the law of cause and effect.

Kundalini Yoga: This is an energetic practice that requires the practitioner to continuously move through the poses to awaken the body, mind, and spirit. It is usually rapid and repetitive.

Mantra: A phrase, word, or sound that is repeated while you are meditating to bring focus, awareness, and presence to the practice.

Mudra: Mudra refers to the positions of your hands during your practice, which brings about connection, focus, and concentration. The most well-known is Anjali, where you press your palms together at your heart and Jnana, where you form a circle with your forefinger and thumb.

Namaste: Namaste is commonly expressed at the end of a yoga class while bowing the head and pressing your palms together at your heart. It is a respectful greeting that honors the other person.

Om: A very common mantra that is chanted at the end or beginning of a yoga class and has many different meanings. Om is said to be the original sound and point of all creation.

Parasympathetic Nervous System (PNS): One of the parts of your body's nervous system that controls how your body reacts and calms down after a stressful situation.

Power Yoga: This was created in the 80s as a more athletic form of yoga. These practices are individualized because they follow a teacher's particular style instead of a set of asanas.

Prana: This is the energy and force of life.

Pranayama: These are specific breathing exercises that aim to clear any obstacles in our body, either physical or emotional. The aim is to free the breath or *prana*.

Sanskrit: The language of ancient India and Hinduism.

Satsang: A gathering to hear an experienced yoga teacher speak and share knowledge.

Shanti: Spoken mantra that is chanted in class and means peace.

Surya Namaskar: A very popular sequence of asanas or sun salutations.

Sympathetic Nervous System (SNS): One of the parts of your body's nervous system that controls your unconscious actions, such as your fight or flight response.

Unilateral: One-sided.

Upanishad: The ancient yogi texts that were written in India around c. 800 BCE. The text focuses on the religious and philosophical nature of yoga.

Vinyasa: These are postures or poses that are strung together to form a flow. The movement is always linked to breathing.

Yamas: These are five moral, ethical, and societal principles for those practicing yoga.

Yang Yoga: This style of yoga is rhythmic and repetitive. It is also more energetic and is commonly used to build strength and improve fitness.

Yin Yoga: This yoga is performed slowly, and the poses are usually held for a longer length of time. It is a more passive form of yoga compared to yang yoga.

Yoga Nidra: A calm relaxed state that is known as *yogic sleep*. It is described as the state between being conscious and awake and being asleep.

Yoga Sutras: An ancient Indian text that describes the philosophy of yoga.

Yogi: A person who practices yoga.

Thank you for your recent purchase of this book.

I hope you love it! I'd kindly like to ask you to leave a brief review on Amazon. Reviews aren't easy to come by, but they have a profound impact. So, we would be incredibly thankful if you could just take a minute to leave a quick review, even if it's just a sentence or two!

You can do it simply just clicking this link:
https://www.amazon.com/review/create-review?asin=B0B3W6XK6C

Thank you so much for taking the time to leave a short review. We are very appreciative as your review makes a difference. This will help me keep up with your needs and also help others like you to find this helpful book. Review or not, we still love you!!

You can subscribe on my page and as a Thank you I'll give you a Free copy of my secrets of incredible weight loss e-book.

Simply subscribe by clicking this link:
www.jannahadams.com

References

Aerobic activity of older adults. (n.d.). Wayne State University.https://cphs.wayne.edu/occupationa l-therapy/resources/exercise_-_aerobic_activity_for_older_adults_1.pdf

Australian Seniors. (2017, February 14). *Benefits of yoga for seniors*. https://www.seniors.com.au/funeral-insurance/discover/benefits-of-yoga-for-seniors

Baiera, V. (2021, June 15). *Benefits of chair yoga for seniors - reduce pain and improve health*. Step2Health. https://step2health.com/blogs/news/benefits-of-chair-yoga-for-seniors

Basavaraddi, I. V. (2015, April 23). *Yoga: Its origin, history, and development*. Ministry of External Affairs. https://www.mea.gov.in/search-result.htm?25096/Yoga:_su_origen

Bernier, J. (2020, August 12). *The 5 golden rules of yogic breathing*. beYogi. https://beyogi.com/5-golden-rules-yogic-breathing/

Britton, A., Hardy, R., Kuh, D., Deanfield, J., Charakida, M., & Bell, S. (2016). Twenty-year trajectories of alcohol consumption during midlife and atherosclerotic thickening in early old age: Findings from two British population cohort studies. *BMC Medicine, 14*(111). https://doi.org/10.1186/s12916-016-0656-9

Burgin, T. (2021, June 22). *79 yoga words and Sanskrit terms to know for class.* Yoga Basics. https://www.yogabasics.com/connect/yoga-blog/sanskrit-yoga-words/

Carney, R. M., & Freedland, K. E. (2016). *Depression and coronary heart disease.* Nature Reviews Cardiology, 14(3), 145–155. https://doi.org/10.1038/nrcardio.2016.181

Centers for Disease Control and Prevention. (n.d.-a). *How much physical activity do older adults need?* https://www.cdc.gov/physicalactivity/basics/older_adults/index.htm

Centers for Disease Control and Prevention. (n.d.-b). *Tips for better sleep.*https://www.cdc.gov/sleep/about_sleep/s

leep_hygiene.html#:~:text=Make%20sure%20y
our%20bedroom%20is

Centers for Disease Control and Prevention. (2021,
    November 16). *Fast facts about arthritis.*
    https://www.cdc.gov/arthritis/basics/arthritis-
    fast-facts.html

Cornwell, B., & Laumann, E. O. (2015). The health
    benefits of network growth: New evidence from
    a national survey of older adults. *Social Science &
    Medicine,* *125,* 94–106.
    https://doi.org/10.1016/j.socscimed.2013.09.0
    11

Damodaran, A., Malathi, A., Patil, N., Shah, N.,
    Suryavansihi, & Marathe, S. (2002). Therapeutic
    potential of yoga practices in modifying
    cardiovascular risk profile middle-aged aged men
    and women. *The Journal of the Association of
    Physicians of India,* *50*(5), 633–640.
    https://pubmed.ncbi.nlm.nih.gov/12186115/

Division of Agriculture. (n.d.). *How to get started with chair
    yoga.* University of Arkansas.
    https://www.uaex.uada.edu/life-skills-
    wellness/health/physical-activity-
    resources/chair-yoga.aspx

Drah, H. (2020, December 18). *34 life-altering yoga statistics & facts for a balanced 2022.* MedAlertHelp. https://medalerthelp.org/blog/yoga-statistics/

Drugs.com. (2023, January 23). *Aging.* https://www.drugs.com/health-guide/aging.html

Elaine Gavalas. (2013, September 17). *YOGA SEATED TRIANGLE POSE (chair yoga) - yoga therapy [Video].* Youtube. https://www.youtube.com/watch?v=W9yFtJO9scc

Emanuel, E. J. (2014, September 18). *Why I hope to die at 75.* The Atlantic. https://www.theatlantic.com/magazine/archive/2014/10/why-i-hope-to-die-at-75/379329/

Fiske, A., Wetherell, J. L., & Gatz, M. (2009). Depression in Older Adults. *Annual Review of Clinical Psychology, 5*(1), 363–389. https://doi.org/10.1146/annurev.clinpsy.032408.153621

Fitnessfit. (n.d.). *This is what happens if you don't warm up before exercising.* https://fitnessfit.com.au/warming-up-before-exercising/

Fitzpatrick, K., & Burford, M. (2021, July 29). *The ultimate guide to yoga lingo.* Greatist. https://greatist.com/fitness/ultimate-guide-yoga-lingo

Freytag, C. (2022, February 4). *20-minute strength training workout for seniors.* Verywell Fit. https://www.verywellfit.com/20-minute-senior-weight-training-workout-3498676

Friedman, H. A. (2017, May 30). *Healthspan is more important than lifespan, so why don't more people know about it?* Institute for Public Health. https://publichealth.wustl.edu/heatlhspan-is-more-important-than-lifespan-so-why-dont-more-people-know-about-it/

Galic, B. (2023, January 23). *92 yoga statistics you need to know.* LIVESTRONG.COM. https://www.livestrong.com/article/13768863-yoga-statistics/

Gaspari Nutrition. (2019, September 1). *What are the major muscle groups?* https://gasparinutrition.com/blogs/fitness-facts/what-are-the-major-muscle-groups

Green, N. (2015, April 4). *The breath is boss, the breath is yoga.* Ekhart Yoga.

https://www.ekhartyoga.com/articles/practice/the-breath-is-boss-the-breath-is-yoga

Harvard Health Publishing. (2020, July 20). *Exercise 101: Don't skip the warm-up or cool-down.* https://www.health.harvard.edu/staying-healthy/exercise-101-dont-skip-the-warm-up-or-cool-down

Harvard Pilgrim Health Care. (n.d.). *5 of the biggest myths about aging.* The Boston Globe. https://sponsored.bostonglobe.com/harvard-pilgrim/biggest-aging-myths/

Jain, S. C., Uppal, A., Bhatnagar, S. O. D., & Talukdar, B. (1993). A study of response pattern of non-insulin dependent diabetics to yoga therapy. *Diabetes Research and Clinical Practice, 19*(1), 69–74. https://doi.org/10.1016/0168-8227(93)90146-v

Jaul, E., & Barron, J. (2017). Age-Related diseases and clinical and public health implications for the 85 years old and overpopulation. *Frontiers in Public Health, 5*(335). https://doi.org/10.3389/fpubh.2017.00335

Jha, P., Ramasundarahettige, C., Landsman, V., Rostron, B., Thun, M., Anderson, R. N., McAfee, T., & Peto, R. (2013). 21st-century hazards of smoking and benefits of cessation in the United States. *The New England Journal of Medicine, 368*(4), 341–350. https://doi.org/10.1056/NEJMsa1211128

Kamb, S. (2023, January 12). *Warm up properly: The 15 best dynamic warm up exercises & routines to prevent injury.* Nerd Fitness. https://www.nerdfitness.com/blog/warm-up/

Kovar, E. (2015, June 18). *Chair yoga poses | 7 poses for better balance.* Ace. https://www.acefitness.org/resources/everyone/blog/5478/chair-yoga-poses-7-poses-for-better-balance/

Kristal, A. R, Littman, A. J, Benitez, D., & White E. (2005). Yoga practice is associated with attenuated weight gain in healthy, middle-aged men and women. *National Library of Medicine*, 11(4), 28–33. https://pubmed.ncbi.nlm.nih.gov/16053119/

Kutcher, M. *(2021, June 6). Balance exercises for seniors.* More Life Health. https://morelifehealth.com/articles/intermediate-balance-exercises-for-seniors

Lindberg, S. (2020, March 10). *Chair exercises for seniors.* Healthline.

https://www.healthline.com/health/chair-exercises-for-seniors#leg-routine

Martins, F. (n.d.). *Chair yoga precautions*. Yoga Teacher Training Blog. https://www.yoga-teacher-training.org/2012/02/06/chair-yoga-precautions/

Martins, F. (2022, November 3). *Chair yoga precautions*. Aura Wellness Center. https://aurawellnesscenter.com/2022/11/03/chair-yoga-precautions/

Mayo Clinic Staff. (2019). *Exercise: When to check with your doctor first*. Mayo Clinic. https://www.mayoclinic.org/healthy-lifestyle/fitness/in-depth/exercise/art-20047414

McEwen, B. S. (2017). Neurobiological and systemic effects of chronic stress. *Chronic Stress, 1*(1), 247054701769232. https://doi.org/10.1177/2470547017692328

Mills, M.. (2020, January 28). *22 chair exercises for seniors & how to get started*. Vive Health. https://www.vivehealth.com/blogs/resources/chair-exercises-for-

seniors#Chair%2520Core%2520Exercises%252
0for%2520Seniors

Moffat, S. D., An, Y., Resnick, S. M., Diamond, M. P., & Ferrucci, L. (2019). Longitudinal change in cortisol levels across the adult life span. *The Journals of Gerontology: Series A, 75*(2), 394–400. https://doi.org/10.1093/gerona/gly279

National Centre for Complementary and Integrative Health. (2015, November 4). *Americans who practice Yoga report better wellness, and health behaviors.* National Institutes of Health (NIH). https://www.nih.gov/news-events/news-releases/americans-who-practice-yoga-report-better-wellness-health-behaviors

National Institute of Aging. (n.d.-a). *A good night's sleep.* https://www.nia.nih.gov/health/good-nights-sleep#aging

National Institute on Aging. (n.d.-b). *How older adults can get started with exercise.*

https://www.nia.nih.gov/health/how-older-adults-can-get-started-exercise

National Institute on Aging. (n.d.-c). *10 myths about aging.* https://www.nia.nih.gov/health/10-myths-about-aging

National Institute on Aging. (n.d.-d). *What is dementia? Symptoms, types, and diagnosis.* https://www.nia.nih.gov/health/what-is-dementia

National Institute on Aging. (2019, April 23). *Social isolation, loneliness in older people pose health risks.* https://www.nia.nih.gov/news/social-isolation-loneliness-older-people-pose-health-risks

Pain Doctor. (2019, September 16). *Chair yoga for seniors and those with limited mobility: 12 poses to try.* https://paindoctor.com/chair-yoga-for-seniors/

Paturel, A. (2016, November). *Yoga poses for your 50s, 60s and 70s - and beyond.* AARP. https://www.aarp.org/health/healthy-living/info-11-2013/health-benefits-of-yoga.html

Pietrzak, R. H., Zhu, Y., Slade, M. D., Qi, Q., Krystal, J. H., Southwick, S. M., & Levy, B. R. (2016).

Association between negative age stereotypes accelerated cellular aging: Evidence from two cohorts of older adults. *Journal of the American Geriatrics Society, 64*(11), e228–e230. https://doi.org/10.1111/jgs.14452

Pizer, A. (2021, December 7). *Yoga equipment guide for beginners.* Verywell Fit. https://www.verywellfit.com/yoga-equipment-guide-for-beginners-whats-essential-3566978

Purdie, M. (2022, October 26). *What is a cooldown?.* Verywell Fit. https://www.verywellfit.com/what-is-a-cool-down-3495457

Rethinking Drinking. (n.d.). *What are the U.S. guidelines for drinking?* https://www.rethinkingdrinking.niaaa.nih.gov/How-much-is-too-much/Is-your-drinking-pattern-risky/Drinking-Levels.aspx

Rountree, S. (2022, June 4). *15 health benefits of aging adults that will make you want to start practicing now.* Yoga

Journal.   https://www.yogajournal.com/yoga-101/15-anti-aging-health-benefits-of-yoga/

Sadhguru. (n.d.). *What is yoga? The original meaning of yoga.* Isha.   https://isha.sadhguru.org/yoga/new-to-yoga/what-is-yoga/#point6

Saint-Maurice, P. F., Troiano, R. P., Bassett, D. R., Graubard, B. I., Carlson, S. A., Shiroma, E. J., Fulton, J. E., & Matthews, C. E. (2020). Association of daily step count and step intensity with mortality among US adults. *JAMA, 323*(12), 1151–1160. https://doi.org/10.1001/jama.2020.1382

Schein, C. (2018, September 21). *11 common aging health issues.*   Aegis   Living. https://www.aegisliving.com/resource-center/11-common-aging-health-issues/

Stelter, G. (2020, May 29). *7 yoga poses you can do in a chair.* Healthline. https://www.healthline.com/health/fitness-exercise/chair-yoga-for-seniors#Warrior-I-(Virbhadrasana-I)

Sullivan, E. V., & Pfefferbaum, A. (2019). Brain-behavior relations and effects of aging and common comorbidities in alcohol use disorder:

A   review.   *Neuropsychology,*   *33*(6),   760–780.
https://doi.org/10.1037/neu0000557

The Sunflower Channel. (2019, August 10). *Chair yoga:*
Gentle warm up & short routine [Video]. YouTube.
https://www.youtube.com/watch?v=AjpDXL
Tlb7A

Tangen, C., Cummings, S. W., & Wood, B. (2018).
Human muscle system. In Encyclopædia Britannica.
https://www.britannica.com/science/human-
muscle-system

TED-Ed. (2016, June 9). *Why do our bodies age? - Monica*
Menesini *[Video].* YouTube.
https://www.youtube.com/watch?v=GASaqPv
0t0g

Tomko, J. (2020, August 28). *How bad is it really to skip a*
warm-up? LIVESTRONG.COM.
https://www.livestrong.com/article/13726404-
skipping-warm-up-exercises-effects/

Tomlinson, K. (2015, December 10). *Yoga lingo for*
beginners. Ekhart Yoga.

https://www.ekhartyoga.com/articles/practice/yoga-lingo-for-beginners

Tummee. (n.d.). *Chair seated warm up flow yoga.* https://www.tummee.com/yoga-poses/chair-seated-warm-up-flow

21 chair exercises for seniors: Complete visual guide. (n.d.) California Mobility. https://californiamobility.com/21-chair-exercises-for-seniors-visual-guide/#8_extended_leg_raises

UW Health. (2017, January 2). *Tree pose - modified sequence* [*Video*]. YouTube https://www.youtube.com/watch?v=w8RYbob19a4

WebMD Editorial Contributors. (2021, March 23). *Health issues in older adults.* WebMD. https://www.webmd.com/healthy-aging/health-issues-in-older-adults

Wilson, A. (2015, June 16). *Breathing during yoga poses.* Inner Light Publishers. https://www.inner-light-in.com/2015/07/breathing-during-yoga-poses/

Wishhart, M. (n.d.). *What do people wear to Bikram yoga?* Chron. https://livehealthy.chron.com/people-wear-bikram-yoga-4079.html

World Health Organization. (2017, December 12). *Mental health of older adults.* https://www.who.int/en/news-room/fact-sheets/detail/mental-health-of-older-adults

World Health Organization. (2022, October 1). *Ageing and health.* https://www.who.int/news-room/fact-sheets/detail/ageing-and-health

Yoga for Harmony and Peace. (2020, June 2). *Yoga.* Yoga.ayush.gov.in. https://yoga.ayush.gov.in/blog?q=58

Yoga Seattle. (2022, February 1). *Best yoga chairs for 2022.* Seattle Yoga News. https://seattleyoganews.com/best-yoga-chairs/#Innolife

Yogapedia. (2020, April 23). *Yoga.* In Yogapedia. https://www.yogapedia.com/definition/4/yoga

Image References

Alonso, M. (2021). *Young Asian woman stretching leg on wooden chair [Image]*. Pexels. https://www.pexels.com/photo/young-asian-woman-stretching-leg-on-wooden-chair-7592317/

Aurelius, M. (2021). *Woman practicing yoga [Image]*. Pexels. https://www.pexels.com/photo/woman-practicing-yoga-6787160/

Helvaci, L. (2021). *Woman in orange tank top and black leggings sitting on a wooden chair [Image]*. Pexels. https://www.pexels.com/photo/woman-in-orange-tank-top-and-black-leggings-sitting-on-a-wooden-chair-9787907/

Krukau, Y. (2021b, February 13). *Elderly people exercising [Image]*. Pexels. https://www.pexels.com/

Krukau, Y. (2021). *Elderly people doing jump rope [Image]*. Pexels. https://www.pexels.com/photo/elderly-people-doing-jump-rope-6815737/

Krukau, Y. (2021b, June 22). *Elderly people doing yoga [Image]*. Pexels.

https://www.pexels.com/photo/elderly-people-doing-yoga-8436479/

Pixabay. (2017). *Grilled meat dish served on white plate [Image].* Pexels. https://www.pexels.com/photo/asparagus-barbecue-cuisine-delicious-361184/

Shuraeva, A. (2021). *Photo of an elderly woman and an elderly man exercising [Image].* Pexels. https://www.pexels.com/photo/photo-of-an-elderly-woman-and-an-elderly-man-exercising-8795593/

Shuraeva, A. (2022). *An elderly couple exercising together [Image].* Pexels. https://www.pexels.com/photo/an-elderly-couple-exercising-together-8795577/

Shvets, A. (2020). *An elderly woman workout watch by the fitness coach.* Pexels. https://www.pexels.com/photo/an-elderly-woman-workout-watch-by-the-fitness-coach-4587381/